101 of Surgical Instruments

Margret Liehn · Hannelore Schlautmann

101 of Surgical Instruments

Naming, Recognizing, Handling and Presenting

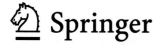 Springer

Margret Liehn
Tating, Germany

Hannelore Schlautmann
Wallenhorst, Germany

This book is a translation of the original German edition „1x1 der chirurgischen Instru-
mente" by Liehn, Margret, published by Springer-Verlag GmbH, DE in 2017. The translation was done with the help of artificial intelligence (machine translation by the service
DeepL.com). A subsequent human revision was done primarily in terms of content, so that
the book will read stylistically differently from a conventional translation. Springer Nature
works continuously to further the development of tools for the production of books and on
the related technologies to support the authors.

ISBN 978-3-662-63631-2   ISBN 978-3-662-63632-9   (eBook)
https://doi.org/10.1007/978-3-662-63632-9

Preface

We are pleased that it has been possible for us to produce the third edition of this book by artificial intelligence. The staffing situation in the individual operating departments has not improved in recent years; work intensification, different duties and less staff complicate the training and education of new employees in the operating room.

Every employee benefits from good induction concepts and comprehensible standards. Despite motivated practice supervisors, however, it is essential to complete the level of knowledge through self-study.

In this edition, we have tried to explain the basics of surgical instruments and to deepen them with illustrations.

Thank you for the feedback we continue to receive from OR staff for this book to help navigate the initially "impenetrable jungle" of instruments.

We would like to thank Aesculap AG for providing us with many illustrations for the third edition as well as all Ethicon and Storz for allowing us to use special illustrations.

Furthermore, colleagues have willingly supported us with their expertise and answered all questions that arose from practical experience. In particular, we would like to mention Mr. Klaus Dieter Harmel (Niels Stensen Kliniken, Marienhospital Osnabrück, Head of CSSD) and Ms. Manuela Junker (Niels Stensen Kliniken, Marienhospital Osnabrück).

Mrs. Gabriele Frank (Rheinböllen) supported us with research concerning the history of the instruments.

This book would not have been possible without the support of Springer-Verlag, in particular Dr. Ulrike Niesel and Ms. Sarah Busch and Ms. Ulrike Hartmann.

We hope that we have once again succeeded in providing operating theatre staff with a book that will help them to recognize and correctly use the instruments and thus contribute to their capability to carry out this demanding and interesting profession even more professionally and for the benefit of our patients.

Margret Liehn
Tating, Germany

Hannelore Schlautmann
Wallenhorst, Germany
Spring 2021

Contents

Introduction

Contents

© Springer-Verlag GmbH Germany, part of Springer Nature 2022
M. Liehn, H. Schlautmann, *101 of Surgical Instruments*, https://doi.org/10.1007/978-3-662-63632-9_1

An essential part of the work of the operating theatre nurses consists, in addition to the important activity of non-sterile theatre assistance, usually referred to as circulating nurse, of taking over handling and presenting the instruments during surgical operations.

In return, it can be expected that the nursing staff in the operating theatre know the required instruments and their intended use and can correctly prepare the surgical instruments for each planned operation. Precise preoperative diagnostics make it possible to plan surgical procedures accurately. As a result, preparation can usually be defined in standards and can be readily referenced.

With the preparation of the containers the work of the scrub nurse starts in cooperation with the circulation nurse.

Before the other materials for an operation are prepared under sterile conditions, the sterility of the instrument containers is checked and it is determined whether all the required instruments are present. The documentation labels of the containers are either stuck on a prepared piece of paper for the patient documentation or, better, read with a scanner for the digital patient record.

> ❯ All materials used in and on the patient must be prepared, documented and approved for use by the OR staff.

Scrub nurses can be expected to name the instruments, to provide them in a correct manner, and to hand them to the operator in such a way that immediate use is possible. In this connection it is desirable that the scrub nurse should be sufficiently familiar with the course of the procedure to know in advance which instrument will be required. Insight into the surgical field - in order to recognize the anatomical structures - helps to draw conclusions about the progress of the surgical intervention. In this way, the required instruments can be handed over - at best without being asked.

Each instrument has been manufactured for its specific use, and it is possible to identify the use for which it is suited on the basis of certain criterias. The names of the instruments result either from their function, their inventor, their manufacturer, but also from their shape, the organ they are used for, or their characteristic. Since in some clinics individual instruments have also been given their own names, it is difficult, especially for new employees, to properly name these instruments. However, if the instrument's function can be deduced from its shape, this task becomes more comprehensible.

Especially in difficult surgical situations, it is expected that the correct instrument can be used immediately without naming it.

The reprocessing criteria must be known, even if the reprocessing is usually carried out in the central sterile supply department (CSSD) because responsible handling of the valuable instruments requires this knowledge. They represent a considerable asset, which has to be preserved for a long time.

> ❯ We can only implement without problems what we understand and know. Only those who know what they are doing and strive to maintain an overview in every situation can work efficiently.

For the most part, instruments are provided in subject-specifically equipped trays in the container and completed by individual instruments as required. Each tray is equipped according to the house standard and this standard is binding. It must be borne in mind that the weight of the containers must be easily manageable by each employee.

This book is intended to provide insight into the manufacture of instruments, to explain the naming and use of each instrument, to give advice on the preparation of instrument tables and to help to learn how to present instruments without complications and stress, in order to make surgical assistance a success.

Only a few instruments can be mentioned by way of example, and the names do not always correspond to those given in the catalogue, especially as different manufacturers use different names.

Continuous technical innovation leads to the production of multifunctional instruments and mechatronic systems, which cannot be covered here.

1.1 History of Instrument Manufacture

Hannelore Schlautmann

The history of instruments goes hand in hand with the development of surgery.

Since the beginning of human history, men and women with healing skills have sought to rid their fellow human beings of disease and treat injuries. Using all their senses - sight, touch, taste, smell and hearing - they have tried to identify and treat illnesses, often with the aid of instruments. Stone Age bone finds show healed fractures that were probably stabilized with splints. Skull trepanations were successfully performed, as evidenced by healed drill rims on skull finds.

In the Pharaonic empires, extensive medical knowledge was already available; around 2500 years ago, more than 200 different instruments for performing operations were already known. The **Edwin-Smith Papyrus** and the **Papyrus Ebers** date from around 1550 BC. They contain the first descriptions and instructions for wound treatment and wound healing. The writings of **Archimatheus** from Salerno from 1100 BC are among the earliest sets of rules for medical conduct.

The Amazons of Greek mythology had a breast amputated in order to be able to better pursue their warcraft with bow and arrow, so there must have been instruments and surgical methods for this. Instruments were made of stone and bone. Archaeological findings show that plant fibres, animal sinews and the biting tools of large ants were used to close wounds in various cultures as early as 500 BC.

Hippocrates of Kos was born around 460 BC on the Greek island of Kos and died around 370 BC in Larisa. He is considered the most famous physician of antiquity and the founder of medicine as a science. He is credited with 61 writings, but these were written between 400 BC and 100 AD - it is unclear which of these were written by himself. Hippocrates explains diseases with an imbalance of the four bodily fluids (blood, phlegm, yellow and black bile) and suggests a change of lifestyle, diet, medicines and surgical interventions such as bloodletting and cupping to cure them.

After the fall of the Greek Empire and at the beginning of the rise of the Roman Empire, more and more medical knowledge reached Rome with Greek doctors. Greeks like **Heliodorus** and **Japyx** brought it to great influence. During Rome's countless campaigns, physicians acquired great knowledge; military physicians developed into the best surgeons. The motto of the Roman commanders was: "The best surgeons to the best legions". An eight-volume encyclopaedia "De medicina", written by the Roman physician **Cornelius Aulus Celsus** (around 25 to 50 AD), reveals a high level of knowledge among surgeons.

Excavations from Pompeii give us an insight into the history of instruments. The city was buried under a six-meter-high layer of ash, lava and debris during an eruption of Mount Vesuvius on August 24, 79 BC. In 1771, during excavations in a house there, a large package of surgical instruments was found. Metal instruments, not unlike those in use today, were already being used here. The first double-ended instruments also date from Roman times.

But it was not only in the West that medicine developed - doctors also researched and healed in the Orient, and the art of healing developed all the better the more injuries were caused by wars. We know from early Arabic writings that shortly after the introduction of Islam, medical knowledge was already at a high level - there were hospitals, doctors and nurses who had to prove they had training and had to follow certain standards. In Cairo, for example, in the Qalawun Hospital, a hospital for almost 8000 patients, cataract operations with sharpened metal tubes were already being performed in the early Middle Ages.

During the Middle Ages, medicine in Europe incorporated the experience of the ancient natural physicians and the medical knowledge of classical antiquity (around 200 AD, **Galenus of Pergamon** made a decisive contribution to a renaissance of the teachings of Hippocrates). Above all, however, it was the unconditional faith in saints that was believed to cure diseases.

Medical knowledge reached Europe with the Crusaders, but its dissemination was hindered by ecclesiastical dogmas and decrees. In the eyes of their representatives, church doctrine contradicted research and experimentation on humans. Thus, the dissection of corpses was forbidden in order to protect the human soul, and specific learning about the interrelationships in the human body was made difficult as a result. The result was scholastic medicine (theoretical textbook medicine) with its theoretically highly educated, but practically only partially operational and successful doctors, who, however, enjoyed high social prestige.

Far below them in the social hierarchy were wound doctors and bathers, who acquired practical knowledge during the frequent wars, as well as barbers and blacksmiths, who provided the common people with surgical procedures such as tooth extractions and abscess splitting. The least respected were the executioners, who, however, often had excellent anatomical knowledge due to their occupation.

In the course of time, however, the Church's resistance loosened, research was carried out and discoveries were made - evidence of which can be found, among many others, in the anatomical drawings of **Leonardo da Vinci** (1452–1519) and numerous surgical textbooks written in the 16th and 17th centuries.

Instruments for use by doctors were made by armourers and cutlers. While natural materials such as bones and stones were used in the early history of surgery, bronze was added later in the form of cast and forged bronze. As metal refinement developed, the composition of instruments changed. Brass and copper instruments were followed by forged ones made of ferrous materials, which were protected from corrosion by metallurgical processing - an important requirement when asepsis was introduced. Another requirement, namely to produce instruments that were easy to clean, meant that elaborate ornaments made of ivory, precious stones and precious metals, which had been common before, had to be abandoned.

1

In the nineteenth century, **Ignaz Philipp Semmelweis** (1818–1865) was the first to discover the cause of childbed fever. In his clinic, medical students went directly to the obstetrics ward after dissection hours in the pathology department. There they examined the women in childbed without washing their hands beforehand. Semmelweis suspected this to be connected with the high mortality of the women. He believed that "corpse particles" thus entered the women's organism and caused an infection there. He then introduced thorough hand washing and hand disinfection with chlorine for doctors and students before they were allowed to enter the maternity ward. By this simple measure, he was able to considerably reduce the mortality of women giving birth.

Joseph Lister (1827–1912) noticed that airborne germs caused wound suppuration and introduced disinfection of the entire surgical area, instruments and dressings with carbolic to reduce germ growth. He is considered the founder of antisepsis.

After these groundbreaking discoveries in the field of hygiene and after ether, chloroform and nitrous oxide (1842–1844) were used to successfully combat pain during operations, a rapid development began in the field of surgical techniques and at the same time in the manufacture of instruments.

Medical development in the nineteenth century was shaped by many doctors
- Theodor Billroth (1829–1894)
- Robert Koch (1843–1910)
- Bernhard R. K. v. Langenbeck (1810–1887)
- Robert Liston (1794–1847)
- Cesar Roux (1857–1918)
- Curt Schimmelbusch (1860–1895)
- Ignaz Philipp Semmelweis (1818–1865)
- Joseph Lister (1827–1912)
- Rudolf Virchow (1821–1902)

They developed and helped to design important instruments such as retractors (Langenbeck, Roux), clamps (Billroth) and scissors (Liston) and gave them their names. Even today, these instruments are part of the basic surgical instruments.

In the twentieth century, the advancement of technology also changed surgery. Many technically sophisticated devices made activities easier and more precise.

The development of robots operated by the surgeon changed operations and the tasks of the surgical team. Nevertheless, operations are always performed "by hand" - robots must be controlled, intestinal anastomoses sutured by hand or performed by machine using a stapler. However, this is not possible without surgical preparation by hand. In trauma surgery, saws, hammers and chisels are still used, which certainly look similar to the ancient models.

Surgery and craft, tools of the trade and instruments are always associated with each other in their development and can only be considered together. Like any good craftsman, a surgeon needs manual dexterity, technical understanding and creativity.

In order to work successfully in his profession, every craftsman has individual tools in which he invests a lot of money and which he treats with care. This is especially true in the medical field. There, the selection, use, care and precise knowledge of the instruments are part of the daily routine of all doctors and nurses in the functional area of clinics and medical practices.

With the industrial production of instruments, new job descriptions appeared - from the professions of cutler and precision mechanic, that of the surgical mechanic was created in 1939. He manufactures and maintains medical-surgical and cosmetic instruments, implants and medical devices. Surgical mechanics work in handicraft businesses in the medical technology sector, but also in industrial companies where medical instruments are manufactured (◘ Fig. 1.1).

Direct contact between surgeons and instrument manufacturers is still important because the requirements for surgical instruments are still largely defined by the users. This is how ideas are created from practice for practice. By reviewing and optimizing the instrument containers, a suitable instrument for individual use can be defined and produced in cooperation with the manufacturer.

Today, better and better instruments and equipment allow for ever larger and more complex surgery.

New technologies are opening up new methods - in some procedures, it is already possible to dispense with the cutting components. Thanks to modern imaging techniques, many interventions, e.g. in vascular surgery the aortic aneurysm, are no longer treated surgically with a vascular prosthesis, but by the radiologist with a stent. No surgical instruments are required for this. For the patient, this is a much gentler method that positively influences the healing process.

Pioneers of modern surgical instruments
- Erich Lexer (1867–1937)
- Harvey Cushing (1869–1934)
- Ferdinand Sauerbruch (1875–1951)
- Michael deBakey (1908–2008)
- Denton A. Cooley (1920–2016)

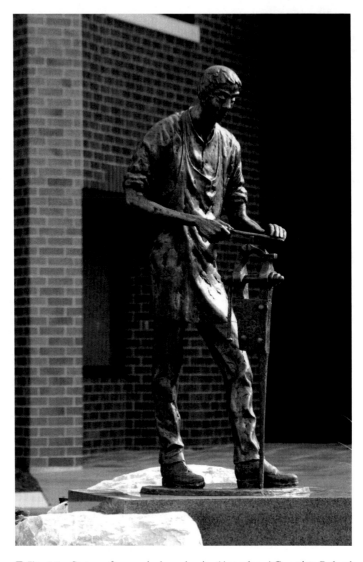

Fig. 1.1 Statue of a surgical mechanic. (Aesculap AG, artist: Roland Martin, with kind permission)

1.1.1 **The Wound Closure**

Historically, suturing a wound is a very old treatment method and has always been a concern of doctors. As early as 500 BC, wounds were closed with plant fibres, linen threads or animal sinews. In ancient times and the Middle Ages, people used gut strings for musical instruments and as bowstrings but also to close open wounds. In the sixteenth century, catgut, a thread made from the intestines of sheep, was used. Important progress is made in the further development of threads and needles.

In 1908, the first industrial sutures are manufactured by the B. Braun company.

But it was not until the 1970s that the first braided (multiple filaments), fully absorbable, synthetic suture material was developed, and from 1981 to 1984 a monofilament (single filament) synthetic absorbable suture material was also developed. Today, modern synthetic materials are used almost exclusively.

Synthetic adhesives are produced for skin closure, which glue the tissue together and no longer require piercing the cutis with needles. This is becoming increasingly important in plastic, reconstructive surgery, breast surgery and facial surgery. Adhesives save operating time, suture material (foreign bodies) and have a good cosmetic result.

1.2 Materials of Surgical Instruments

Hannelore Schlautmann

On the world market there is a very large supply of stainless steel grades made from a wide variety of alloys. However, only very few of them meet the high requirements for the manufacture of medical and, in particular, surgical instruments. After all, these instruments are subjected to the highest stresses during use and must perform their tasks flawlessly. To ensure this, high-quality standards apply to the production of surgical instruments.

For example, forceps and clamps are expected to retain their elasticity for a long time and chisels and scalpels should be capable of cutting over the long term and not break. During use, the instruments are exposed to a wide variety of chemical (body fluids, cleaning agents and disinfectants), physical (pressure, lever forces) and thermal (disinfection, steam sterilization 134 °C, high-frequency surgery approx. 1000 °C) influences. The challenges this poses for manufacturers in the search for and development of appropriate materials and manufacturing processes are enormous.

Surgical instruments are manufactured from a variety of metals, metal alloys, plastics and ceramic materials. All these materials are adapted to their respective intended use according to the latest state of technology and research and are certified according to different national standards (▶ Sect. 1.3). Plastics and hard fabrics are used, for example, as hammer handles, on-ear funnels, endoscopes, as insulation on instruments, as adhesives and sealing materials. Ceramic materials are used in implants in trauma surgery and orthopaedics, glass in optics. The majority of materials, however, are various metals.

1

All are subject to international standards and are specially processed and alloyed according to their use, i.e. they contain metals, carbon or other chemical substances in varying proportions. These additives affect, among other things, their strength, elasticity, rust resistance, electrical conductivity and, of course - their price.

The most commonly used steels for instruments and implants are chromium, nickel and molybdenum, which are responsible for rust and corrosion resistance, titanium but also copper is processed. Copper is used in jaws of some needle holders, but also as an additive in steel joints. Titanium is increasingly used in various alloys because of its special hardness, but also because it hardly causes allergies. When processed, titanium has a matt, light-metallic shiny appearance. Instruments and implants made of titanium are light but strong, corrosion-resistant, ductile and slightly magnetic. However, due to the complicated manufacturing process, titanium parts are about 10 times more expensive than comparable steel parts.

Titanium was discovered in 1791, but its industrial production has only been possible on a large scale since 1940. Titanium alloys are often characterized according to the US standard ASTM (American Society for Testing and Materials) comparable to other national standards.

Titanium
- Pure titanium has material number 3.7034.
- The materials 3.7164 and 3.7165 are titanium alloys whose main alloying elements are aluminium and vanadium.
- The most common titanium alloy on the market is Ti6Al4V.

Titanium is used as an implant in dentistry (cheaper than gold, lighter than steel), orthopaedics (as a joint replacement and osteosynthesis material), neurosurgery (more favourable magnetic properties than steel) and microsurgical instruments (does not lose its delicate tips even in autoclaves). Titanium coating is also used for instruments in plastic surgery and cardiac surgery. The instruments are coated with titanium after grinding in order to maintain the special sharpness longer.

In addition to the classification by material number, each steel is also given a short name based on what the steel is to be used for. It is also common to classify steels according to their chemical composition.

Chemical abbreviations for material abbreviations
- Cr - Chrome
- Mn - Manganese
- Mo - Molybdenum
- Ni - Nickel

- N - Nitrogen
- S - Sulfur
- V - Vanadium
- Ti - Titanium

An example for understanding:

The steel with the material number 1.4301 and the short name X5CrNi1810 is the well-known V2A steel:
- The X stands for high-alloy steel (stainless steel),
- the number 5 for the carbon content, here 5%,
- the letters Cr and Ni for the chemical elements chromium and nickel,
- the number combination 1810 for the amount of 18% chromium and 10% nickel added to the pig iron.

The terms **austenitic**, **ferritic** and **martensitic** steel indicate the stress and strain of the corresponding types of steel - for example, martensitic steels are used in the manufacture of, among other things, scissors, knives and cutting pliers because of their hardness, while austenitic steels are specially heat-treated, which gives them resistance to alkalis and acids, for example. Austenitic steel is used to make containers, trays, retractors and the like.

Some instruments have a special hard metal insert made of a chrome-tungsten alloy, which increases durability and functionality due to its hardness. These instruments are identified by a gold handle (▶ Sect. 1.4).

Implant steels are used for steel implants (e.g. endoprosthesis, plates, screws), but also for the instruments used to prepare the implantation, such as drills or milling cutters. Here, too, pure austenitic steels are used in particular, as implants have to meet special requirements. They must be able to withstand high dynamic loads, must not be magnetizable and must not offer any surface for tissue fluids to attack.

1.3 Norms and Standardisation

Hannelore Schlautmann

Norms are the basis for standardization and quality assurance. It is not an invention of modern times - bricks were already standardized in ancient Egypt, the Romans had standard dimensions for their water pipes and in the fifteenth century standardized individual parts were used in shipbuilding in the Republic of Venice.

To ensure that the various high-grade steels used in industry are of comparable quality, they are subject to a basic standard.

1

Testing procedures of several institutes ensures the comparability of the different worldwide standards, i.e. DIN standard 17,442 for instrument steel in the Federal Republic of Germany is the same standard as in Singapore, provided that a manufacturer has undergone the German standardization procedure. There are different standards applying to stainless steel for surgical implants, which is subjected to different tests than that for general instruments.

On a European and international level there are other organisations which have made it their task to standardise and thus make raw materials, manufacturing processes, finished products and applications comparable - on a European level this is EN (European Standard) and on an international level it is ISO (International Standards Organisation).

When purchasing new goods, the ISO numbers provide clear information on materials, design and test requirements, among other things. They thus facilitate, for example, technical comparison at an international level. Each standard must be reviewed every 5 years. Depending on the result, the standard is confirmed, revised or withdrawn.

1.4 Surface Finish

Hannelore Schlautmann

To ensure that the instruments do not dazzle the surgeon during the intervention due to the bright operating light, the surfaces of the instruments are matted. After an instrument has been manufactured, it is given this matt finish either by sandblasting or matt brushing. During sandblasting, the polished surface of the instrument is dented by the bombardment with tiny glass beads and thus becomes matt.

Gold-plated rings at the working end of an instrument indicate that this instrument has a hard metal insert (▶ Sect. 1.2) in the instrument jaws. This plating is made of pure gold. This prevents corrosion, e.g. due to chemical reactions during reprocessing.

1.5 Handling of the Instruments by the Scrub Nurse

Margret Liehn

The instrumentation of a surgical procedure requires a great deal of knowledge. The OR nurse is familiar with the anatomy as well as the planned course of the operation. From the anatomical position, the organ structure and the planned operation, it is often possible to determine which instruments in particular are needed, how they should be shaped and what special corrugation inside the jaws is required.

In order to be able to hand out instruments quickly, purposefully and with foresight, the situs must be visible and the instruments must be clearly structured and accessible.

Beforehand, it is necessary to practice working with both hands equally, because one hand is used to hand an instrument, while the other hand is used to pick up the one previously used.

Most people have one preferred hand and the other, mostly the left, has to learn many things first. The following exercises can help to train the second hand (the information applies to right-handers):

— Brush your teeth with your left hand.
— Guide the knife while eating with the left hand,
— also eat the soup with a spoon in the left hand.
— Use of scissors with the left hand, even right-handed scissors can be used with the left (!),
— brush the hair with your left hand.

There are many more examples that could help to train the second hand to facilitate hand movements with the left hand during the assistance of surgical interventions. It is important not to practice using the second hand effectively only during the presentation.

1.6 Basic Rules

Margret Liehn

Every employee must know the contents of the instrument containers; if necessary, a visit to the CSSD during the training period can help. In any case, lists are showing which instruments are kept in the container trays and in what numbers.

Instruments must be prepared for the planned operation in a standardized manner (▶ Chap. 5). The set-up of the instrument table, as well as the side tables, is bindingly regulated for each employee via standards, which facilitates intraoperative replacement, which can and must be possible at any time.

Basic trays contain the instruments that are always needed, so the contents vary in the specific surgical departments. In addition, there are special trays, individually packaged additional instruments and disposable materials.

All instruments that are required in a standardized manner for the planned operation are ready on the instrument table, everything that may be required is on the additional table. The trays are placed on one or more additional tables and only what is needed is removed. If the planning changes intraoperatively, the scrub nurse must prepare instruments during the ongoing procedure and request new instrument containers if necessary.

In the operating departments, it is handled differently whether the scrub nurse may reach into the clean tray with the used gloves during the operation in order to prepare additionally required instruments, or whether a sponge forceps must be prepared for this purpose. Since all instruments prepared for the operation must be prepared in the same way in the CSSD (▶ Sect. 7.3), both are possible.

The functions, as well as the names of the instruments, are known because everyone on the surgical team must speak the same language so that there are no avoidable delays or even errors. Many instruments look deceptively similar and yet have different names and tasks. Knowledge of the shape and profiles often makes the task clear, yet one surgeon may use the same instrument differently from another. Provided that this goes hand in hand with the purpose of the instrument, this is not a problem. In addition, there are the preferences of individual surgeons for certain familiar tools, which should be taken into account.

In the best case, the required instrument is presented without prompting by the surgeon, but always swiftly and in such a way that the surgeon can immediately grasp the rings or handles of the instrument without having to reach around. For this purpose, the instrument must be watched until it arrives in the surgeon's hand. If the surgeon can work immediately without turning the instrument, the instrument was correctly positioned.

This requires some practice because the surgeon is usually standing opposite the scrub nurse and it is difficult at first to understand how the instrument must then be presented in order to be immediately usable.

Surgical instruments

Contents

© Springer-Verlag GmbH Germany, part of Springer Nature 2022
M. Liehn, H. Schlautmann, *101 of Surgical Instruments*, https://doi.org/10.1007/978-3-662-63632-9_2

2

Surgical instruments are manufactured for a specific purpose, which is evident from the construction and design of the instrument. Instruments are matt metallic, black and/or have a golden handle as identification, which indicates that a carbide insert has been inserted in the front of the working part (▶ Chap. 1). These instruments do not need to be refinished and the manufacturers give a longer warranty on such instruments.

We distinguish between cutting, grasping, clamping, and retracting instruments. Some of them look very similar on the outside, but the function is made clear by the different corrugation at the jaws.

The naming of the instruments has different reasons. Sometimes it depends on the inventor, for example, **Kocher clamp**, or on their intended use, such as **dissecting scissors**. If the manufacturer is considered the name giver, a name of the surgeon who modified the instrument according to his ideas may be added, for example, **abdominal retractor by Fritsch**.

In order to ensure consistency of terminology in the following, it must be possible to name the individual parts of the instrument correctly. This also makes it easier to describe an error when requesting a repair or to provide explanations on how to hand the instrument when training new employees.

In addition to the assistance, the scrub nurse is also responsible for ensuring that the intended purpose of the instrument is observed in order to preserve its functionality.

2.1 Design and Intended Use

An instrument is designed in such a way that it is optimal for the user as well as for the application. Regardless of the size of the hand that guides the instrument, it must lie well in the hand, be of optimal weight, and be easy to guide. Depending on the purpose, it can be cut, held, clamped, locked or kept closed with pressure.

In addition to the purpose of the instrument, it must be possible to reprocess it without any problems (▶ Chap. 7). Depending on the intended use, instruments must be able to be closed and, if necessary, fixed in the closed position (locking). Either the surgeon closes the instrument only by hand, for example, with micro-instruments and some needle holders, or there is a ratchet option with which the working parts can be kept closed without effort. In this case the OR staff must know which instrument may be closed with how many grids of the ratchet. (For preparation in the CSSD the instrument must be open, for sterilization grids may not be closed under any circumstances; ▶ Chap. 7)

An instrument consists of one, two or more parts. Two-part instruments are connected either by springs or screws or olives in the jaw.

We distinguish the following parts of an instrument:

- The **rings** that hold the surgeon's fingers. They can be of the same size or different sizes to accommodate one or more fingers.
- The **branches**, the part of the instrument between ring and jaw.
- The **grip surfaces** on which an instrument is held. This part of the instrument is roughened or grooved to provide a good grip for the surgeon's fingers.
- The **lock** or **ratchet** is the device that allows an instrument to be closed and the closure to be kept. This lock has different grids, the closing of which is discussed accordingly with the instruments in the following text.
- The **working part**, or mouth or jaws, which grasps and holds the corresponding tissue or material.

Some instruments are equipped with elastic working parts that allow them to reopen automatically. This makes it easier for the surgeon to feel how much pressure the instrument must be used with.

Basic Instruments

Contents

© Springer-Verlag GmbH Germany, part of Springer Nature 2022
M. Liehn, H. Schlautmann, *101 of Surgical Instruments*, https://doi.org/10.1007/978-3-662-63632-9_3

The basic instrument set includes the instruments that are needed for every operation. These always include scalpel, scissors and forceps (anatomical blunt as well as surgical sharp), short retractors (blunt and sharp) as well as clamps and needle holders. The structure, task and handling of each basic instrument are discussed in detail.

3.1 General Instruments

In every surgical department, the basically used instruments vary in size and number. Basic instruments are always prepared and special instruments are added depending on the planned operation. In principle, the departmental standard applies here, so no claim to completeness can be made in the following.

3.1.1 Scalpels

To open the skin, a scalpel is needed. It consists of a handle and a blade. It does not matter whether the scalpel is a disposable instrument with a plastic handle or a reusable handle in which the blade is clamped. The designation is based on the layer to be cut, e.g. skin knife (◘ Fig. 3.1), or on the shape of the blade, e.g. stabbing scalpel. The different sizes are coded with numbers.

The most important thing about a scalpel is the sharpness of the blade. Cutting through the cutis wears down a sharply ground blade to the point that other tissue layers can no longer be sharply cut with this blade. Due to the large, bulbous shape of the skin knife, the scalpel is easy to guide and cuts quickly and evenly. In order to cut through deeper tissue layers, the blade must be smaller so that the area to be cut can be seen (◘ Fig. 3.2).

Another option is the stab scalpel, which is triangular and pointed. It can be used to make incisions for drainage or as access for scissors, cannulas, trocars or similar (◘ Fig. 3.3).

In this connection the amputation knife should also be mentioned, which is a reusable instrument and is used to cut through the soft tissues in an amputation. This knife (named after **Virchow**, **Langenbeck** or **Liston**) must always be sharpened and is handed in exactly the same way as a scalpel, although the size of the instrument sometimes makes it difficult to remove after use (◘ Fig. 3.4).

In ENT or oral and maxillofacial surgery (OMS), as well as in microsurgery, the handles for the scalpel blade can be

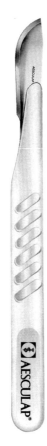

Fig. 3.1 Scalpel skin. (Aesculap AG, with kind permission)

bayonet-shaped or angular-bent in order to make an incision in a confined space and not obstruct the view with the surgeon's hand (**Fig. 3.5**). Reusable blades are also available here, e.g. for paracentesis, for the tonsils or the septum.

■ **Handling**

The disposable blades are usually packaged in a single aluminum foil. To ensure sterility, the scrub nurse must accept the blade with a blunt clamp and then wait until the circulation nurse has checked in backlight whether the packaging was without damage, only after the "OK" of the "circulator" the blade is usable.

The presenting of a scalpel (**Fig. 3.6**) to the surgeon should be seen from two points of view. Firstly, the surgeon should get the instrument and be able to work immediately. Secondly, it is very important to give the instrument to the surgeon in such a way that there is no risk of injury to the staff. For this purpose, the scalpel is grasped from above so that the

3

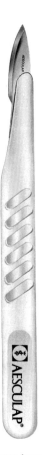

◻ Fig. 3.2   Scalpel for deeper tissue layers. (Aesculap AG, with kind permission)

blade points downwards towards the patient. The surgeon has two options for guiding the instrument, either he grips the blade from above and then cuts, or he grips the scalpel like a pen and cuts as if he were trying to write (◻ Figs. 3.7 and ◻ 3.8).

It should be noted that the blade never comes into contact with the hand of the instrument user, whether the knife is handed or removed after use.

The surgeon returns the knife after use and the OR nurse grasps it again from above without coming into contact with the sharp side of the blade. It should be noted here whether the surgeon turns the scalpel over to protect the nurse and hands it over with the handle first. In this case, care must also be taken not to graze anyone with the blade when removing the scalpel.

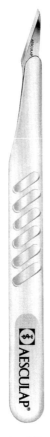

Fig. 3.3 Stitch scalpel. (Aesculap AG, with kind permission)

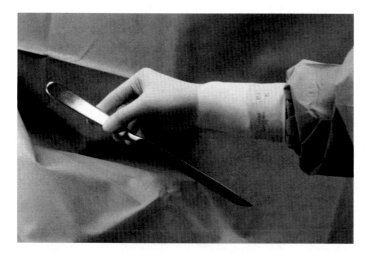

Fig. 3.4 Handling of an amputation knife. (Photo by Margret Liehn)

3

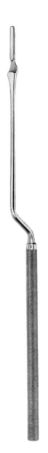

◘ Fig. 3.5 Bayonet scalpel handle for a disposable blade. (Fa. Aesculap AG, with kind permission)

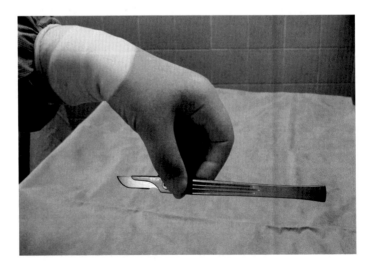

◘ Fig. 3.6 Presenting a scalpel. (Photo by Margret Liehn)

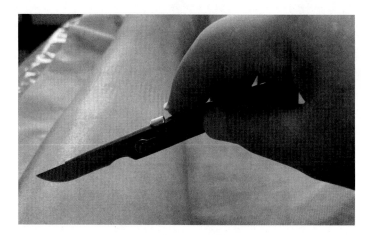

☐ Fig. 3.7 Guiding a scalpel 1. (Photo by Margret Liehn)

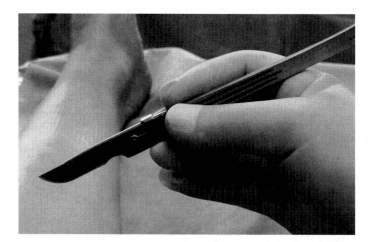

☐ Fig. 3.8 Guiding a scalpel 2. (Photo by Margret Liehn)

Another problem is the removal of the disposable blades from the knife handle, which involves an increased risk of injury. The blades may only be grasped with a coarse blunt clamp in order to be removed from the handle, because blood and secretion cause the blade to stick in the anchoring and can only be removed by applying skill and force. Using the fingers the danger of injury would be too high and thus the removal without clamp is obsolete.

3.1.2 **Tweezers**

Forceps belong to the basic instrument set as well as to the special instrument set. They grasp the tissue to be cut, prepared or sutured and are profiled accordingly on the inner surface of the jaws. To hold the tissue, they must be able to grip, and to hold the vessel for haemostasis by means of high-frequency current. The surgeon needs them while holding the needle or the scissors in his other hand, to grip tissue or to grasp the needle, the forceps are the extension of his fingers.

Tweezers consist of two halves that are pressed together when they hold the tissue and they spring back into their original position when the pressure of the fingers is released. To ensure that they lie well in the hand and do not slip even when gloves are wet, they have a roughened or grooved gripping surface on the outside of their legs.

Some models have a pin on one leg that fits into a recess in the other leg. This prevents the jaws from shifting against each other when too much pressure is applied, which makes it impossible to grip with a precise fit (in surgical jargon, this is referred to as "squinting" tweezers). Tungsten carbide inserts are also used for tweezers, in which case the marking is again a golden grip. As a rule, the jaw profiles are cross-grooved, which allows a firm grip with relatively little pressure.

Depending on the tissue to be gripped, the following three types of forceps are distinguished.

■ **Surgical Sharp Forceps**

Surgical tissue forceps are sharp and have several teeth on both sides that interlock when squeezed, i.e. the number of teeth must be unpaired (◘ Fig. 3.9). When tissue is grasped, this allows the tissue to be held firmly. The number of teeth varies. Behind the tooth, the gripping surface is often still cross-grooved, this allows additional hold of the tissue. They are used to hold subcutaneous fatty tissue or to grasp coarse structures such as muscle or fascia.

The size and number of teeth are determined by the tissue to be grasped. The **Adson forceps** is considered an example of delicate surgical forceps (◘ Fig. 3.10) and is used for delicate structures on the face, neck and e.g. the dura (these delicate forceps are also available as an anatomical dissecting version, see below).

To obtain tissue for histological examination, forceps with an annular opening in the tip of the forceps legs and surgical serration are often used (◘ Fig. 3.11).

The length and shape of the required forceps is adapted to the surgical site. There are an infinite number of variants. In the parlance of the operating room, use is made of coarse short or long fine, **Adson** or similar short names.

■ **Anatomical Dissecting Tissue Forceps**

Anatomical dissecting tissue forceps are blunt and transversely grooved at the front of the working part (◘ Figs. 3.12 and

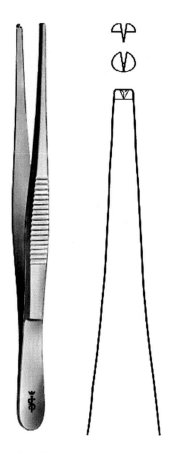

◘ Fig. 3.9 Surgical tissue forceps with a sketch of the teeth. (Fa. Aesculap AG, with kind permission)

3.13). When tissue is held with them, the two halves of the forceps must be strongly pressed together. This squeezes the structure of the grasped material and is therefore not suitable for delicate vessels. However, there are finely tapered anatomical forceps that make it possible to grasp intestinal mucosa, for example, without much pressure and without causing trauma. They thus offer an alternative to atraumatic forceps in visceral surgery. They are available in coarse short, long fine, angled, curved.

Long, fine anatomical forceps are often used for the application of high-frequency (HF) current for haemostasis (see below). Forceps whose legs are coated with an insulating layer can also be used here, which prevents the HF current from being dissipated too early via the forceps legs, as it should only act at the tip of the instrument.

Tweezers that pass bipolar high-frequency current are also insulated and metallic only at the tips. The cable to the current generator is connected directly to the forceps. During use by

3

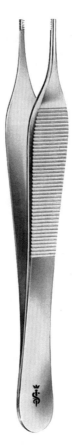

▣ Fig. 3.10 Sharp tissue forceps according to Adson-Brown. (Aesculap AG, with kind permission)

the surgeon, the cable of the forceps must be held tension-free with the other hand of the scrub nurse (▣ Fig. 3.14).

■ **Atraumatic Dissecting Forceps**
Atraumatic forceps are also blunt but are different in profile inside. They can be longitudinally serrated or also have a cross serration. This profile allows grasping without destroying and is therefore used in vascular or intestinal surgery.

Atraumatic forceps with a parallel longitudinal striation in straight or curved form are named after **Cushing**, **De Bakey** (▣ Fig. 3.15) or **Cooley.**

Atraumatic tweezers according to **Cooley** have a more pronounced profile, but also a longitudinal groove with graining around the central groove (▣ Fig. 3.16).

Cross serrated is also considered atraumatic, an example being **Cushing**'s forceps (▣ Fig. 3.17).

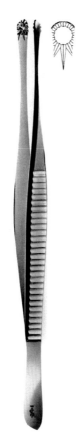

◘ Fig. 3.11 Surgical grasping forceps, Russian model. (Aesculap AG, with kind permission)

Forceps with a lateral angle or curved tip are used in vascular surgery and/or neurosurgery.

Bayonet-shaped forceps, e.g. according to **Gruenwald** (◘ Fig. 3.18), or angled-bent forceps according to **Troeltsch** (◘ Fig. 3.19) are used in the neurosurgery, ENT or OMS departments.

Coagulation forceps form a further subgroup. Any forceps can be used for the application of monopolar current, but fine anatomical forceps are preferred (see above). It should be noted that the current flows through the entire length of the forceps and contact must only be made with the tissue to be coagulated. In surgical jargon, they are often simply called "current" forceps.

When using forceps that are insulated on both legs, contact of the legs with body tissue is safe. Only the jaw ends are made of bare steel, the legs are covered with a plastic layer that does not conduct electricity. Thus, the current is only

3

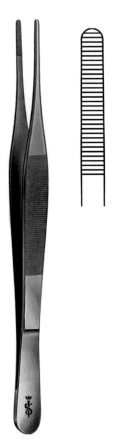

◘ Fig. 3.12 Anatomical Adson dissecting tissue forceps. (Aesculap AG, with kind permission)

applied to both tips of the forceps. When preparing the instruments, it is important to check that the insulating layer is undamaged.

When using **bipolar current**, the current flows into the forceps via a suitable bipolar cable the two tips form the two circuit poles. The current is triggered either by means of a foot switch or via the forceps, which trigger the current flow when both tips of the forceps are in contact with the tissue.

■ **Handling**

Straight forceps are grasped by the scrub nurse at the bottom of the working ends and placed upright in the surgeon's hand. As a rule, the surgeon needs the forceps in addition to the scissors or needle holder, so this instrument usually belongs in the surgeon's left hand (◘ Fig. 3.20).

Experienced scrub nurses can grasp the forceps between the little and ring finger when handing over the needle holder, for example, and by turning the hand immediately after hand-

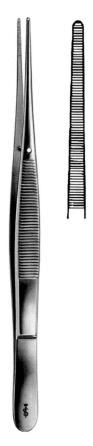

◘ Fig. 3.13 Anatomical dissecting tissue Cushing's forceps. (Aesculap AG, with kind permission)

ing over the needle holder, transfer the forceps to the surgeons other hand. This leaves the other hand free to remove a used instrument (◘ Fig. 3.21).

Angled-bent forceps as well as bayonet-shaped forceps are presented in such a way that the upper angle of the forceps points downwards towards the patient (◘ Fig. 3.22). This is important when working under the microscope, because the surgeon cannot turn the forceps in one hand if the application was not correct but must look away from the microscope to grasp the instrument correctly.

The scrub nurse knows which forceps are suitable for which tissue. The passing of forceps to the scissors or needle holder is done without being asked and immediately after the instrument has been passed to the other hand.

❯ The OR theatre nurse should know whether the surgeon is right- or left-handed, because this determines the position of the scissors in the nurses hand.

3

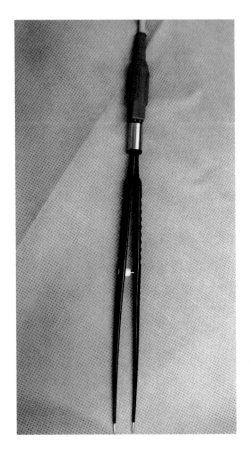

◘ Fig. 3.14 Dissecting forceps for bipolar current. (Photo by Margret Liehn)

3.1.3 **Shears**

Another tissue-cutting instrument besides the scalpel are the scissors. They are one of the most important instruments and can be used for sharp severing, dissection and cutting of various materials. Depending on the depth of the body, the handles are long, curved, angled, and the cutting blades have different curvatures and are ground differently. Working on the surface, the short scissors models are important and in depth, the instrument must be longer. Some scissors are also characterized by a golden handle, carbide blades have a special precision grinding, which does not wear out quickly.

A pair of scissors consists of two parts and three sections. The **handle sections** are either ring-shaped to accommodate the thumb and middle or ring finger, or the handle is spring-loaded and the surface is roughened on the outside, as with micro-scissors, so that the holding hand does not slip off the handle, there is a safe grip.

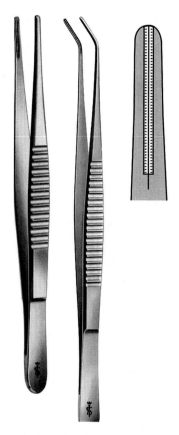

◘ Fig. 3.15 Atraumatic dissecting forceps according to De Bakey, straight and angled. (Aesculap AG, with kind permission)

The connection of the two scissor parts is a screw (▶ Chap. 2); by this the opening and closing of the instrument is made possible. The two cutting parts are called **blades**. They are either both rounded at the end, both pointed, or one blade blunt, one sharply ground. The blade is usually bevelled towards the cutting edge.

The working part of a pair of scissors is either straight, bent or angled according to its application. The bend can be to the right or left, up or down. In order to determine in case of doubt which way the bend of a pair of scissors is pointing, they are placed on a table in such a way that the screw head is visible, which connects the two working parts.

The names of the scissors result from their field of application or correspond to the "inventor".

The most common **dissecting scissors** have slightly rounded blades. When dissecting in depth, one blade is not visible, and therefore it should be blunt, so that it does not cause injury to the surrounding area. On the blade, cutting edge and backside

3

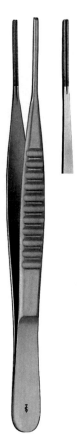

◘ Fig. 3.16   Atraumatic forceps according to Cooley. (Aesculap AG, with kind permission)

are different. Pointed ends of the blades are found on micro-scissors and vascular scissors as well as on very fine dissecting scissors.

If one blade is ground smooth and one is serrated, the scissors are often used as **thread scissors,** as they do not slip off the end of the thread and cut reliably.

The **Metzenbaum** dissecting scissors are the most common scissors in surgery, as they can be used for dissecting many tissues. They are available in all lengths, with carbide blades (golden handle) and without. Their blades are straight or curved, both rounded at the front. It can be used to prepare almost any tissue (◘ Fig. 3.23).

A finer pair of dissecting scissors is, for example, the **Reynolds** scissors (◘ Fig. 3.24), the blades of which are pointed at the tip. In many departments these scissors are called **Wittenstein, Jameson** or **Stevens scissors**. They are used for the preparation of nerves and vessels or in facial surgery.

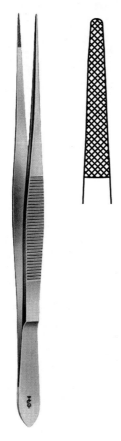

◘ Fig. 3.17 Atraumatic forceps according to Cushing. (Aesculap AG, with kind permission)

If the scissors are straight in the branches and in the blades, they are used to sever lumina that are to be prepared for anastomosis (◘ Fig. 3.25).

Some scissors have a flattened knob on one blade (◘ Fig. 3.26). This blade is used to protect the underlying tissue. For example, it is used to cut the dura mater so as not to injure the underlying brain, or it is used to open a luminal organ, such as the salivary duct or gall duct.

The bending of the blades should be selected depending on the tissue layer when in use. Slightly curved scissors are suitable for exposing superimposed layers, slightly curved organs or for dissecting different structures. The more circular the organ being dissected, the more pronounced the curvature of the blade.

Accordingly, each surgical discipline has different curved scissors (▶ Sect. 4.4). Angled scissors are used in biliary tract surgery and in vascular surgery. The angulation is given in

3

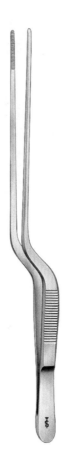

■ **Fig. 3.18**   Bayonet dissecting forceps according to Gruenwald. (Aesculap AG, with kind permission)

degrees. The **Potts de Martell** angled scissors can be used to cut the gall duct or a vein or artery very accurately and without injury to surrounding tissue, or to widen the stab incision of a hollow organ by inserting one blade of the scissors into the lumen after a stab incision and widening it with a straight cut (■ Fig. 3.27).

In OR parlance, these scissors are often just called Potts scissors or angle scissors. This form is also named after **Diethrich**, **Potts Smith**, **De Bakey** and others. In ENT or OMS, angled-bent scissors are used to prevent the surgeon's hand from obstructing the field of vision during narrow accesses, e.g. in the area of the nose.

Micro-scissors are straight or bayonet-shaped; here too, the principle applies that the surgeons hand is not visible in the field of vision of the microscope. In microscissors, the individual blades are spring-loaded (▶ Sect. 4.7).

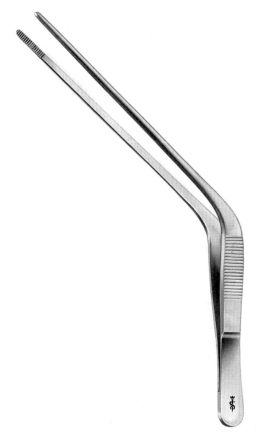

◘ Fig. 3.19   Angled-bent forceps according to Troeltsch. (Aesculap AG, with kind permission)

The size and fineness of the scissors must always be adapted to the material to be cut. A fine vessel cannot be cut with thread scissors, but the reverse is also not possible. If coarse material is cut with scissors that are too fine, the cut suffers and the scissors are dull for the next use and must be reground or replaced.

For cutting coarse materials, **Cooper**'s scissors are one of the best known; they can be used to cut sutures superficially or to cut dressing material intraoperatively (◘ Fig. 3.28).

Comparable are the **Mayo** or **Lexer** scissors, which look similar and are intended for the same use.

The rib shears are used in thoracic surgery, and the individual scissor models are often named after their designer or inventor. They are very strong in order to be able to cut through the bone and usually angled in the cutting blade in order to guide them around the rib and specifically only cut through the bone.

3

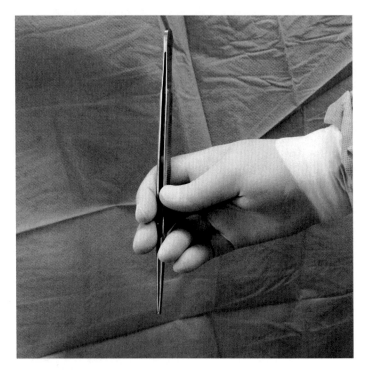

◻ **Fig. 3.20** Presenting of straight forceps. (Photo by Margret Liehn)

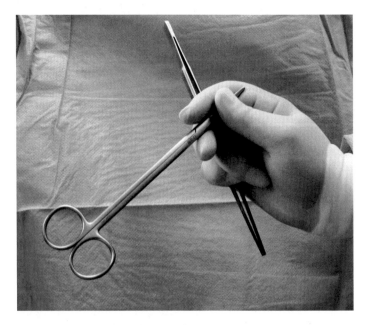

◻ **Fig. 3.21** Presenting scissors and tweezers with one hand. (Photo by Margret Liehn)

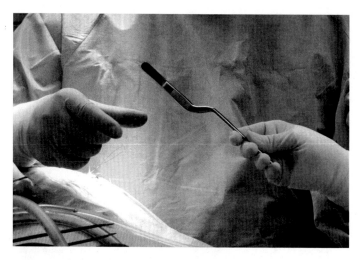

Fig. 3.22 Presenting a bayonet-shaped forceps. (Photo by Margret Liehn)

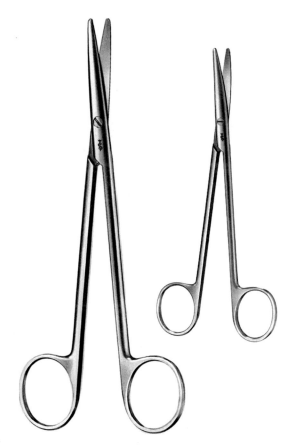

Fig. 3.23 Metzenbaum dissecting scissors. (Aesculap AG, with kind permission)

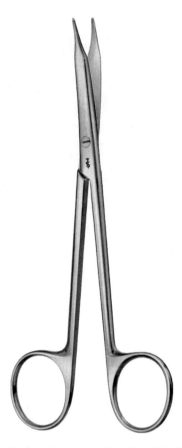

◻ Fig. 3.24   Reynolds dissecting scissors. (Aesculap AG, with kind permission)

Many scissors are named after their function, the proper name is omitted in everyday use, such as the rib shears (**Sauerbruch** ◻ Fig. 3.29, **Brunner** ◻ Fig. 3.30) and the thread scissors (after **Cooper**).

There are scissors for both right-handed and left-handed surgeons, but most surgeons use right-handed scissors, which can also be used by left-handed surgeons.

■ **Bipolar Shears**

Bipolar scissors are connected to the generator with a two-pole cable and coagulate during the cutting process. They are usually shaped like **Metzenbaum** dissecting scissors and are handed accordingly. During presenting, the cable is held tension-free with the other hand.

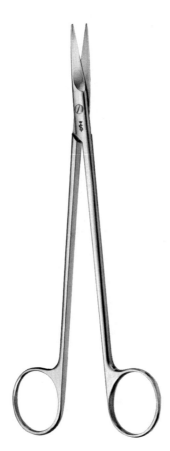

■ **Fig. 3.25** Straight scissors according to Tönnis. (Aesculap AG, with kind permission)

■ **Handling**

The presenting depends on the shape of the scissors and the layer to be prepared or the material to be cut. A pair of scissors is grasped by the scrub nurse at the cutting blades. If the surgeon is standing opposite and the curvature of the blades is above the index finger, the scissors will point downward at the tissue. If the curvature is over the thumb, the bend will point upwards so the surgeon can see which layer the tips of the scissors are in (■ Fig. 3.31).

The rule is that the surgeon should see the tip of the scissors during dissection, this results in the approach. The curvature of the scissors should be adapted to the shape of the organ to be dissected. Shortening of sutures in depth is also done with the tip of the scissors upwards to avoid cutting through the knot.

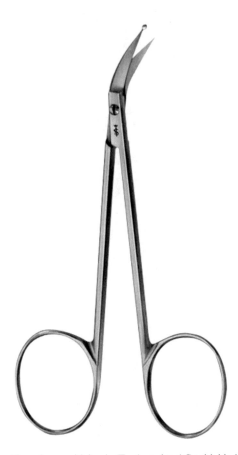

◻ Fig. 3.26   Fine scissors with knob. (Fa. Aesculap AG, with kind permission)

The exception to this is the micro scissors, which are gripped below the spring so that the working parts can be pressed together. When not in use, the spring-type microscissors are open, but like any other instrument, they must be presented closed.

Bayonet-shaped scissors, like forceps, are presented in such a way that the angle of the scissors points downwards towards the patient. Angled scissors, such as those according to **Potts de Martell**, are presented with the cutting surface in the direction of the incision. After a stab incision, a blade is inserted into the opened lumen to then widen the incision.

Rib shears are to be applied in the direction of the rib. Since these scissors have no rings for the surgeon to grasp, the surgeon's hand will grasp both handles of the scissors. In the middle of the handles are two "horns" on which the surgeon's hand can rest, because cutting through a bone requires force.

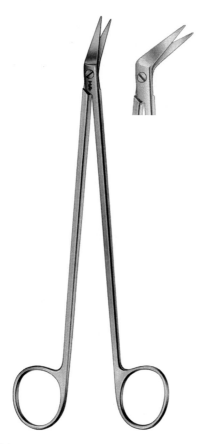

□ Fig. 3.27 Scissors according to Potts de Martell. (Aesculap AG, with kind permission)

Thus, the shape of the instrument depends on the purpose, and the grinding of the blades, too. From this it follows that scissors should cut only the tissue for which they were designed, all other materials destroy the fine grinding and lead to avoidable repair costs.

3.1.4 **Clamps**

Clamps are available in different shapes, but also in different closing mechanisms and profiles. They are available straight, angled, curved, bayonet-shaped and in many other variations in order to adapt their shape to the anatomical conditions.

Clamps grip the tissue or material with both jaws and there are locking grids on the handle that are pressed together and hold until the surgeon releases them. Only then is the tissue released again.

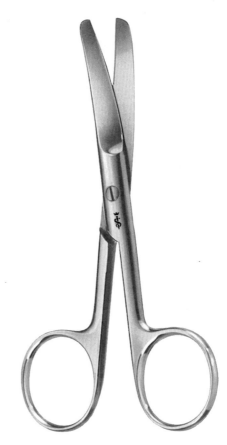

❏ **Fig. 3.28**   Scissors according to Cooper. (Aesculap AG, with kind permission)

As the name suggests, clamps are designed to clamp material, and depending on their intended use, the various grooves already indicated for tweezers apply here:
- dissecting blunt, anatomical,
- atraumatic,
- surgical, sharp.

Depending on the intended use, the shape of the clamp is selected with the appropriate jaw profile. The corresponding jaw profile is available as short-grip as well as long-grip. In addition, surgical sharp clamps have teeth that interlock and are attached to the tip of the jaw surfaces.

In many cases, the cover material is fixed with **towel clamps** (❏ Fig. 3.32). It should be borne in mind that sharp clamps must not be used, as these perforate the cover material and sterility is no longer guaranteed. The towel clamps are called **Backhaus clamps**.

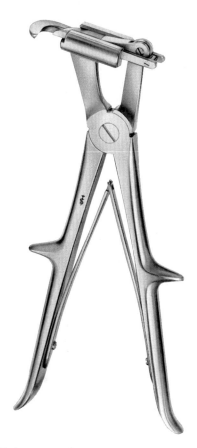

□ Fig. 3.29 Rib shears according to Sauerbruch. (Aesculap AG, with kind permission)

Many clamps are used to clamp materials and work with them in depth. These instruments often have a longitudinal groove in their transverse serration to hold the material without unduly increasing the tension in the jaws. Swabs and very small swabs, for example, are clamped in a dressing forceps to provide a firm grip and to selectively dab up blood or secretions in depth. The instrument is a straight dressing forceps (□ Fig. 3.33) and is used to clamp a swab (□ Fig. 3.34).

When clamping swabs or other materials, it must be remembered that the clamp must be adapted to the size of the swab and the ratchet must not be used up to the last grid in order to avoid unintentional opening of the clamp. Overcoming the last grid leads to the opening and thus to the loss of the swab! The swab is also clamped in such a way that it is possible for the

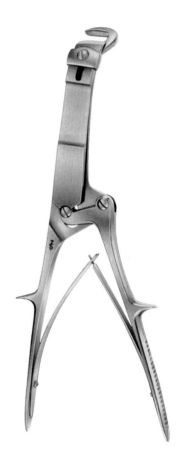

Fig. 3.30 Rib shears according to Brunner. (Aesculap AG, with kind permission)

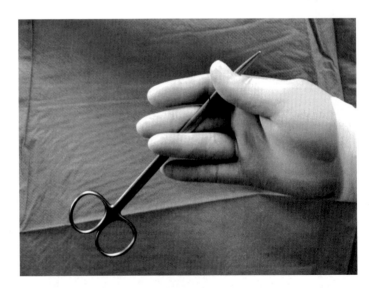

Fig. 3.31 Presentation of curved scissors. The nurse is facing the surgeon, the curved blades are above the thumb, at the tissue the tips of the scissors point upwards. (Photo by Margret Liehn)

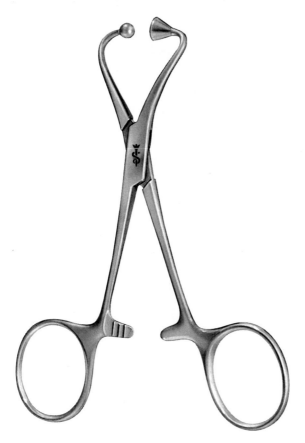

◻ Fig. 3.32 Blunt towel clamp. (Aesculap AG, with kind permission)

surgeon to swab but also to see the surrounding tissue. For this purpose, the swab is rolled up and one third of it is clamped.

The dressing forceps are also available curved. This instrument is used to withdraw drains from an incision, to tunnel subcutaneous fat and to pull through drains, vascular grafts or other implants. Clamps designed for organ grasping are summarized in ▶ Sect. 3.1.5.

■ Traumatic Clamps

Hard grasping clamps grip the material firmly and do not yield in the mouth, so that the tissue is squeezed. These clamps are available as both surgical (sharp) and anatomical (blunt) instruments. As an example, consider the strong **Kocher** surgical **clamp**, which firmly grips the material it grasps (◻ Fig. 3.35). Its teeth give it the characteristic of a surgical clamp. Although they are **in no way** designed to occlude an artery in preparation for anastomosis, they are properly called Kocher's artery clamps. They come in straight and curved forms.

3

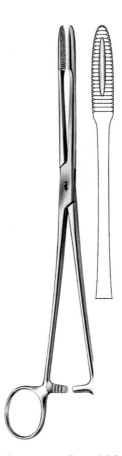

◘ **Fig. 3.33**   Dressing forceps according to Maier. (Aesculap AG, with kind permission)

This clamp is 15 cm long, so it can only be used superficially. It is excellent for clamping threads, rubber reins or other material.

When longer clamps are needed, the **Kocher-Ochsner clamp** is often used. It is constructed in the same way but is altogether longer, it is available up to 35 cm long. Longer and finer, they are called **Halstedt clamps**. This clamp is also available as a surgical and anatomical instrument.

If the clamp is to be smaller and shorter, there is the **Mosquito clamp**, which is available in a blunt and a sharp version (◘ Fig. 3.36). It is similar in design to the Kocher or Péan clamp but is shorter and therefore lighter; if it is to be used as a holding clamp, its weight will not tear the tissue. If the clamps are desired to be still smaller and lighter, they are often called "baby" clamps.

A sharp clamp, the **Mikulicz clamp,** is also chosen to clamp the peritoneal sac for abdominal wall closure. It is also slightly

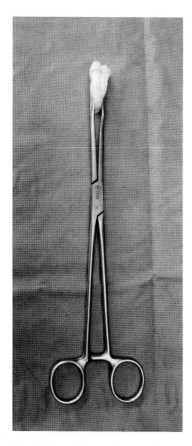

◻ Fig. 3.34 Dressing forceps with a swab. (Photo by Margret Liehn)

curved so as not to hinder the surgeon when suturing. Its small teeth grip the peritoneum so tightly that adaptation for suturing is possible (◻ Fig. 3.37).

The **Péan** haemostatic clamp also grips firmly but does not destroy the surface of the material due to the anatomical grooving (◻ Fig. 3.38). These clamps, like all others, come in various lengths and shapes. They are used to clamp coarse tissue that is not to be damaged by surgical teeth, e.g., thyroid capsule, parenchymal tissue, pleura. Their use is very versatile, but they are not suitable for a vessel for anastomosis preparation, here an atraumatic clamp should be chosen (see below).

Alternative terminal designs comparable to those previously mentioned include those according to **Spencer** or **Crile**.

Hard grasping clamps are not suitable for closing vessels or parts of the intestine if the tissue is still to be used for an anastomosis. They are very well suited as holding clamps for fabric and material.

3

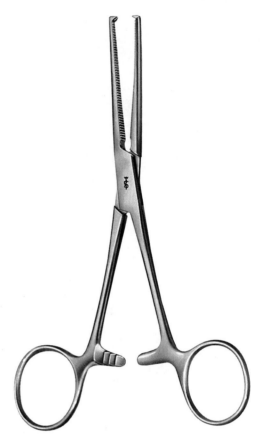

◘ Fig. 3.35   Artery clamp according to Kocher. (Aesculap AG, with kind permission)

■ **Soft Clamps**

If the tissue is only to be closed, but the individual layers are not to be traumatized, soft elastic grasping clamps are used, the jaws of which are designed in such a way that the steel yields resiliently when they are closed.

An example is a soft bowel clamp that closes the bowel but does not traumatize it (◘ Fig. 3.39). This allows blood flow to be briefly interrupted without crushing the vessel walls. This clamp is applied to the portion of the bowel that is to be used to restore intestinal passage. A hard grasping clamp can be applied to the resectate to prevent intestinal contents or tumor cells from escaping.

The use of soft grasping clamps with longitudinal grooving of the working parts will allow the anastomosis to be perfused and necrosis will not occur.

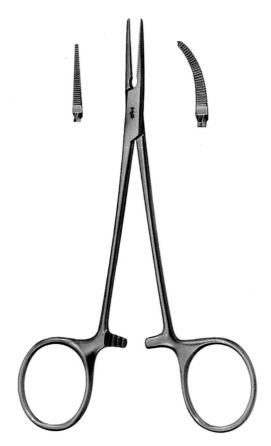

□ Fig. 3.36 Halstedt mosquito clamp. (Aesculap AG, with kind permission)

Similarly designed clamps with the same range of applications are the **Doyen** or **Hartmann** intestinal clamps.

Often, the clamping parts are additionally covered with a tubular bandage to protect the mucosa. Before use, this textile covering must be moistened to avoid sticking to the serosa.

■ **Vascular Clamps/Intestinal Clamps**

In intestinal surgery as well as in vascular surgery, clamps are also required that are not only closed resiliently but also have an atraumatic jaw profile. The arrangement of the groovings and/or serrations prevents traumatization of the sensitive vessel walls. The locking mechanism usually consists of three ratchets so that the closure can be individually adapted to the tissue thickness.

3

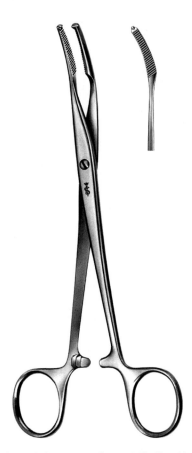

◘ **Fig. 3.37**   Peritoneal clamp according to Mikulicz. (Aesculap AG, with kind permission)

Here the surgeon must consider how far he closes the clamp - the more pressure is applied to the working parts by closing the individual grids - the more forcefully the vessel walls are compressed. Vascular clamps are also curved in such a way that the vessel can be clamped, the bleeding is stopped, but surrounding tissue is not caught. The size of the working part of the instrument is adapted to the lumen and the pressure prevailing in the vessel. The length of the branches corresponds to the depth in the patient's body, so that there are identical clamps in different lengths and especially in different bends of the branches.

The **Satinsky clamp** was originally used in cardiac and vascular surgery, but its shape has also made it popular in abdominal surgery and urology (◘ Fig. 3.40).

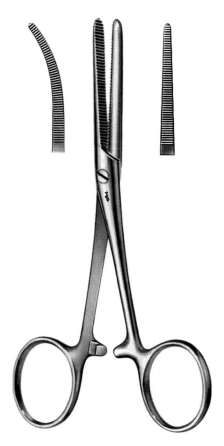

◘ Fig. 3.38 Haemostatic clamp according to Péan. (Aesculap AG, with kind permission)

This clamp has a cross-grooved jaw and is double bent up. This also makes it possible to clamp out part of the lumen. This is particularly necessary in vascular and cardiac surgery if the blood flow is to be partially released while an anastomosis is being sutured. In this case, one "side" of the vessel is clamped in the longitudinal direction, and blood is already flowing through the other "side" to supply the organ in question (this is the process of "clamping out"). It can be used as an arterial clamp, as a venous clamp and also as an intestinal clamp for the part of the intestine to be anastomosed, as well as a renal hilum clamp.

If the jaw profile is longitudinally grooved, the clamp is called a **Price-Thomas clamp** and is also used in thoracic surgery to clamp a bronchus. Atraumatic clamps can be used in intestinal surgery as well as in vascular surgery (▶ Sect. 4.6).

3

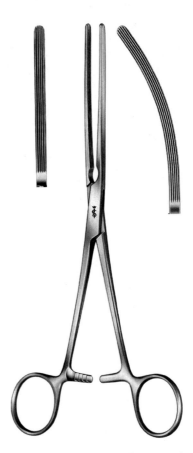

◘ Fig. 3.39   Soft elastic bowel clamp according to Kocher. (Aesculap AG, with kind permission)

■   **Preparation Clamps/Ligation Clamps**

Short-grip, slightly curved instruments with a transversely grooved anatomical jaw surface can be used to bluntly separate tissue structures from one another or to cut off vessels after they have been severed. The bending varies from slightly to strongly curved. The bend is indicated by a number.

The best-known preparation clamp is certainly the **Overholt clamp** (◘ Fig. 3.41). If the instrument is correspondingly smaller and finer for more delicate structures, it is often referred to as a "**baby overholt**". Other similarly constructed instruments with the same range of applications are those according to **Mixter**, **Geissendoerfer** or **Rumel**.

In order to separate tissue structures, two clamps are placed a short distance apart, e.g. on a vessel, and scissors or a scalpel are used to cut between the clamps. A thread is placed around

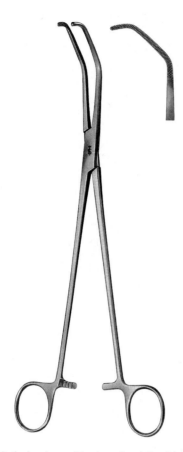

◘ Fig. 3.40 Satinsky clamp. (Fa. Aesculap AG, with kind permission)

the upward bent tip of the clamp and then knotted. After the first knot is tied, the clamp is slowly opened and removed, and then the other knots are tied. If the ligation is done in depth, the ligature thread is clamped in the tip of an Overholt and passed around the positioned clamp (◘ Fig. 3.42).

Another form of preparation can be by means of a guiding probe and a Deschamps (▶ Sect. 3.1.9).

■ Handling

With all clamps it is desirable that the surgeon can reach into the rings of the instrument and that the jaw part points to the tissue layer. Concerning bending or angulation of the branches or/and the jaws, it must be taken into account whether complete or partial clamping is to be performed; accordingly, the bending of the jaw points to the lumen or runs parallel to the lumen.

3

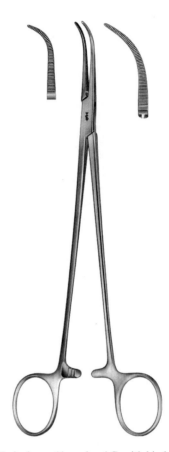

□ **Fig. 3.41**   Overholt clamp. (Aesculap AG, with kind permission)

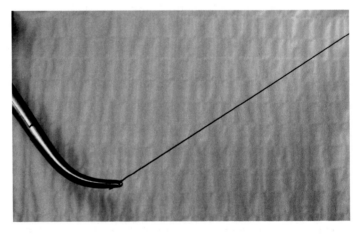

□ **Fig. 3.42**   Overholt clamp with clamped ligature. (Photo by Margret Liehn)

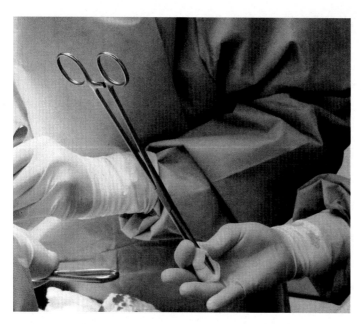

◘ Fig. 3.43 Presenting a dressing forceps with a swab. (Photo by Margret Liehn)

The only exception is the straight dressing forceps with a swab, because here the branches of the instrument are grasped by the surgeon, who does not reach into the rings. The handle is held vertically, grasping the swab with the textile facing the blood (◘ Fig. 3.43).

As a rule, the use of clamps is standardized in surgical departments. Nevertheless, in order to apply the appropriate clamp correctly, the scrub nurse must know which tissue is to be grasped in order to be able to select the appropriate length, bend and jaw profile.

Straight clamps are presented by the nurse grasping the closed clamp at the jaw and placing the rings of the instrument in the surgeon's hand. Curved and angled clamps are presented so that the jaw is placed against the tissue to be clamped without the surgeon's hand obstructing the view of the vessel or bowel.

If it is unclear how the surgeon will apply the clamp, the tip of the instrument must be visible in the operating field, as with the scissors. This means that the surgeon is handed the clamp with the curved tip pointing upwards.

If the nurse is facing the surgeon, the clamp is grasped at the mouth so that the bend wraps around the thumb (◘ Fig. 3.44); if the nurse is standing next to the surgeon, the bend must form around the index finger (◘ Fig. 3.45).

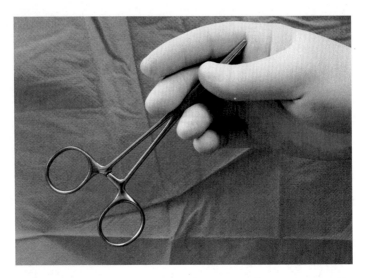

◼ Fig. 3.44   Presenting a clamp, the surgeon standing opposite. (Photo by Margret Liehn)

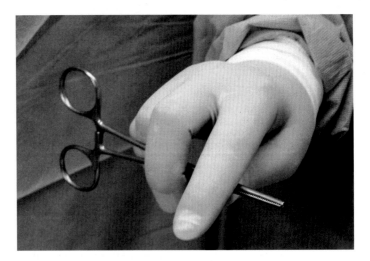

◼ Fig. 3.45   Presenting a clamp, the surgeon standing next to the nurse. (Photo by Margret Liehn)

When ligating structures, it may be necessary for the scrub nurse to hold the end of the suture clamped in an Overholt so that the suture is straightened to be passed in depth around the positioned Overholt clamp, then the suture is released. If the assistant doctor has the opportunity to take over the thread, the end of the thread is handed to the assistant. In such cases, the scrub nurse always has an Overholt armed with a ligature at the ready. It should be noted that the suture also remains on the sterile table and does not hang down under any circumstances in order to ensure sterility.

Clamps come in such a wide variety that it is impossible to mention them all. Every employee in the operating theatre must know the clamps with the designation that is common and be able to recognize from the serration for which they were designed.

In addition to the above-mentioned clamps, there are forceps specially developed for particular tissues, such as parenchymatous tissue, for serosa or coarse tissue such as the uterus, as well as for foreign body removal. They are available with a wide variety of jaw profiles, with atraumatic tips or teeth. The most common ones are presented below.

3.1.5 Organ Grasping Forceps

In order to be able to grasp certain organs firmly, there are corresponding instruments. They are often named after the organ they are intended to grasp, such as the gallbladder grasping forceps or the lung grasping forceps.

These forceps are often round, oval or triangular fenestrated, in order to be able to indicate to the surgeon at any time the state of perfusion of the grasped organ. The striation of the jaws depends on the desire for acceptable trauma. The gallbladder is usually removed when it is grasped, so anatomic striation is not problematic. The lung parenchyma, after it has been grasped, is released again if necessary and must continue to be well perfused, so that atraumatic striation must be used here, because it should fix securely without destroying tissue supply with blood.

In many departments there are different names for the instruments, often shortened variations of the original name (◘ Figs. 3.46 and 3.47). Some structures can only be held with toothed grasping forceps because they are so coarse that forceps without teeth could not hold them firmly. Sharp grasping forceps are then used, either pointed like the hooked forceps according to **Schröder** (▶ Sect. 4.4), or with two to four teeth that interlock sharply, like the hooked forceps according to **Museux** (◘ Fig. 3.48).

If the forceps has only about five small teeth and is wide in the mouth like the grip forceps according to **Allis** (◘ Fig. 3.49), it can be used, for example, to hold the intestine open before a stapler is inserted. To clamp the stomach or the lung, the forceps according to **Babcock** can be used, as it can grip muscles

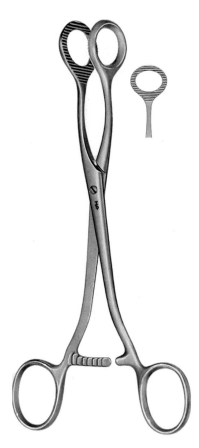

☐ **Fig. 3.46**   Gall bladder grasping forceps according to Doyen (or according to Collin). (Aesculap AG, with kind permission)

better (☐ Fig. 3.50). In the context of MIS (▶ Sect. 4.2), these forceps are popular for fundoplication surgery.

In daily use, it is often difficult to name the individual instruments. In many cases, all triangular fenestrated clamps are referred to as "**Duval**" clamps, but it is important to note the serration, which can be different for instruments with the same name. This can lead to confusion, so always be sure to identify which clamp is specifically needed.

Grasping forceps exist straight, angled or curved and the length of the branches must be adapted to the depth of the situs. 90°-angled clamps with an atraumatic serration are suitable, for example, for depositing the rectum in the lesser pelvis without obstructing the already difficult view, or for depositing the duodenum during gastric resection (☐ Fig. 3.51). 90° clamps are also used in gynecology. The names of these clamps may vary.

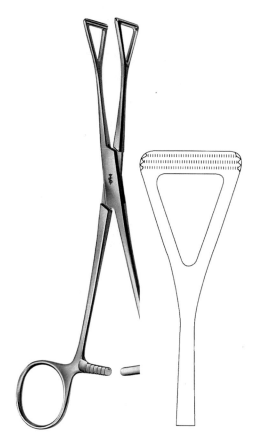

◘ Fig. 3.47 Collin lung grasping forceps. (Aesculap AG, with kind permission)

These or similarly constructed clamps are also known as clamps according to **Götze** or **Wertheim.**

Forceps used to retrieve a stone or foreign body are shaped to match the foreign body (**◘** Fig. 3.52). To remove a splinter, the jaws must be very pointed; to retrieve a stone, the jaws should be spoon-shaped, either fenestrated or closed. In addition, stone grasping forceps often do not have a ratchet, but are closed manually according to the size of the foreign body.

■ **Handling**

Grasping forceps are always applied according to the organ or foreign body and according to the intended use. It must be clear whether an atraumatic, anatomical or surgical sharp profile is required.

Grasping forceps are always handed closed. Straight forceps are grasped at the jaws and the tip is handed diagonally to

3

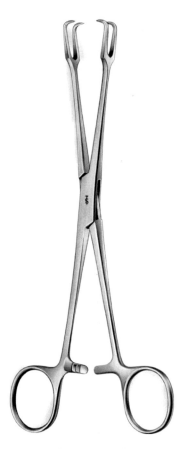

☐ **Fig. 3.48** Organ grasping forceps according to Museux. (Aesculap AG, with kind permission)

the patient, angled and curved forceps so that the tip of the instrument comes to rest over the forefinger of the scrub nurse, presented the surgeon who is standing opposite. The bend of the branches follows the shape of the organ when used.

3.1.6 **Wound Retractors (Hooks)**

In order to be able to keep the surgical area open for the surgeon to reach the target organ, various retracting instruments are needed. These instruments are designed according to the layer that needs to be held aside. They are sharp for the subcutaneous tissue, blunt for muscle and fascia, round for the abdominal wall, wide to hold aside abdominal organs such as the liver while not injuring them, narrow and long if they are

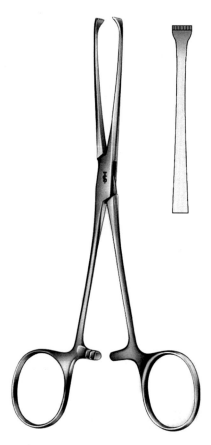

◘ Fig. 3.49 Tissue grasping forceps according to Allis. (Aesculap AG, with kind permission)

to hold aside the urinary bladder in the pelvis, for example. Only if the wound area can be safely held open with the retractors is it safe to use scissors or a scalpel.

Wound retractors have a handle and a shank leading to the working end, also called the blade, which is appropriately rounded or equipped with one to six prongs. The handles either have a grooved surface so that they can be held firmly or they have a fenestrated thickening in the handle where hold is given to the assistant.

Their length corresponds to the surgical site. In the depth of the abdomen long retractors are needed, superficially short variants are sufficient. The most common retractors are presented below. The names of the retractors often refer to famous surgeons, but here too there are many modifications to adapt the instruments to the changing surgical methods.

3

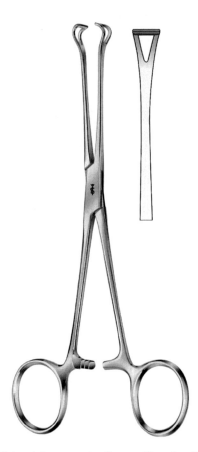

☐ **Fig. 3.50**   Babcock lung grasping forceps. (Aesculap AG, with kind permission)

■ **Examples for Several Retractors**

Sharp or even semi-sharp retractors are used when very strong tissue is to be retained and no sensitive tissue can be injured. The size and number of teeth depend on the size of the skin incision and the amount of tissue to be grasped and lifted. They are usually named based on the sharp teeth: One or 2 prongs, sharp retractors with 2–6 prongs, alternatively they are called **Volkmann retractors.**

Blunt round retractors have flat "blades" and can thus lift structures without injuring them. They are often called eyelid retractor (also vein retractor, ☐ Fig. 3.54), nerve retractor, abdominal retractor or liver retractor, depending on the organ to be lifted. In addition, these retractors often have proper names after their designer, e.g. abdominal retractor according to **Fritsch.**

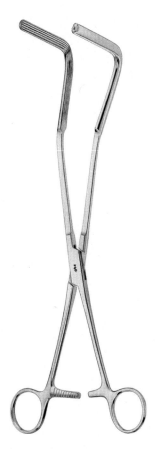

Fig. 3.51 Rectal anastomosis clamp according to Lloyd-Davis. (Aesculap AG, with kind permission)

Exemplary in the basic instrument set there are the **Roux retractors**, which are blunt double-ended retractors that should always be present in pairs (**Fig. 3.53). As a rule, they are available in a set of three in three different sizes, which can be placed one inside the other in the instrument tray. Both ends of the retractor are of different sizes, making them very variable in use. They are often used to push muscles aside.

The **Kocher** vein retractor, which is often used superficially or in neck surgery, should also be mentioned here. It resembles the eyelid retractor (**Fig. 3.54) but is somewhat stronger.

The **Langenbeck** retractor is an angled hook with blades of different widths and lengths (**Fig. 3.55). In the tip, the retractors are additionally slightly bent, which prevents slipping. They are used to carefully hold delicate tissue during a small approach. If the retractor is clearly angled at the front, it

3

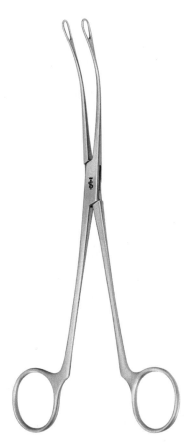

■ **Fig. 3.52** Gall stone forceps according to Blake. (Aesculap AG, with kind permission)

is called a **Langenbeck-Kocher** retractor. Both shapes are available in different lengths and widths.

In the abdominal cavity, the retractors become longer and wider, but remain exclusively blunt (▶ Sect. 4.1).

■ **Handling**

Retractors are prepared in pairs.

The sharp instruments are always placed on the instrument table with the teeth facing upwards so that the cover of the table is not perforated!

When presenting the instrument, it is important to ensure that there is no risk of injury to anyone (■ Fig. 3.56). These retractors are always grasped from above, with the sharp prongs pointing downwards towards the patient, so that the nurse's hand can move away upwards as soon as the surgeon

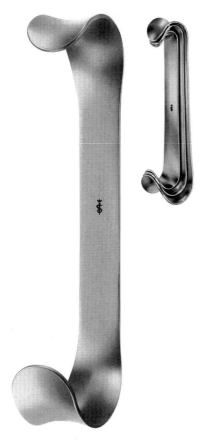

◘ Fig. 3.53 Roux retractor. (Aesculap AG, with kind permission)

has taken the instrument. Removal is also mainly done under safety criteria, as these retractors are very sharp (◘ Fig. 3.57).

When presenting the blunt hooks, the blade points into the surgical site, the hook is either grasped from above or gripped on the blade. The surgeon can easily grasp the handle and place the hook. If the hook is presented to the assistant immediately, the handle must then point towards the assistant and not towards the surgeon.

If the retractors are taken from the surgeon, the sharp retractors must also be grasped from above. Some surgeons take the precaution of turning the retractors around when handing them over, so that the handle points towards the scrub nurse. In this case, it is important to note whether the surgeon grasps the handle from above or from below (if he grasps the handle from below, the sharp prongs can injure the glove or, in the worst case, the hand).

3

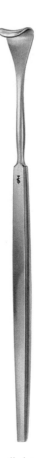

◘ Fig. 3.54 Vein retractor, also called eyelid retractor, according to Mas-ing. (Aesculap AG, with kind permission)

3.1.7 **Self – Retaining Retractors**

In order to keep the situs open when, for example, no assistant is available or is needed for other activities, self-retaining retractors can be used. Either they have a device that allows spreading in differently adjustable positions or they are hooked into frames, in which case they are mostly systems consisting of several parts.

For superficially use retractors are prepared sharp or blunt, depending on the application. After opening the wound, the two blades are inserted and the instrument is fixed in the desired position. As already mentioned, sharp retractors are not used in the deep abdomen (◘ Figs. 3.58, 3.59, 3.60, and 3.61).

Self-retaining retractors are available straight or bent in the handle, or with an adjustable joint, so that variable bending is

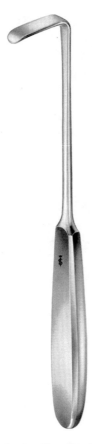

◻ Fig. 3.55 Langenbeck retractor. (Aesculap AG, with kind permission)

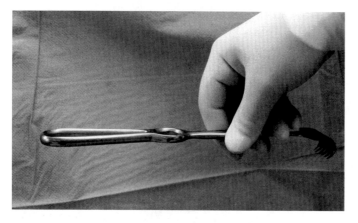

◻ Fig. 3.56 Presenting a sharp retractor. (Photo by Margret Liehn)

3

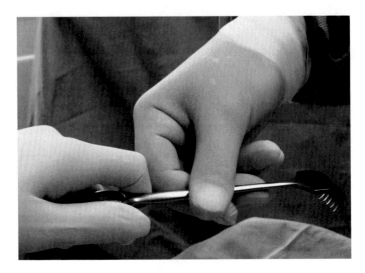

Fig. 3.57 Removing a sharp retractor. (Photo by Margret Liehn)

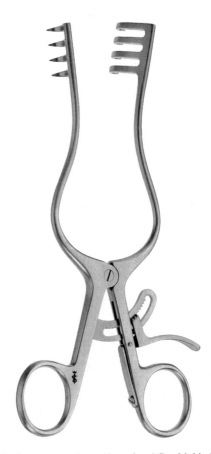

Fig. 3.58 Irwin retractor, sharp. (Aesculap AG, with kind permission)

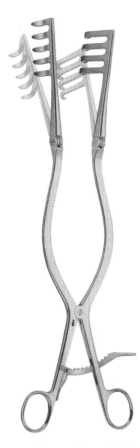

Fig. 3.59 Retractor according to Adson with joint. (Aesculap AG, with kind permission)

possible and the handle of the retractor does not obstruct the surgeon. For some procedures, the blades of the retractor will vary in size as well as shape. Fixation is either by lockable grids or by a locking screw.

There are many self-retaining systems for abdominal surgery, in which either blades of different sizes are hooked into a free ring (**Kirschner frame, Semm holder, Golligher, Balfour** (◘ Fig. 3.63), **Gosset** frame) or a frame system is fixed to the operating table under sterile conditions, into which variable blades can then be hooked.

The self-retaining **Kirschner frame** consists of 5 parts: Frame and 4 blades (◘ Fig. 3.62). The base frame is rigid and the four blades are attached to the base frame according to the extent of the surgical field. The blades are curved to encompass the abdominal wall and keep the surgical field open. The handle of the blades has several small hooks so that they can

3

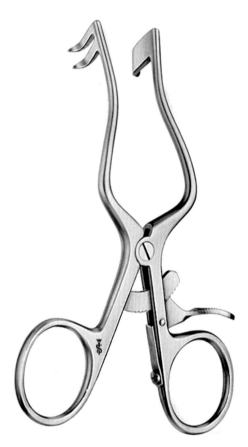

◘ **Fig. 3.60**   Retractor according to Plester. (Aesculap AG, with kind permission)

be clamped to the base frame in tension as needed. If the frame is to be more round, there is a similar system according to **Semm** or **Denis-Brown**.

As an example of universally applicable self-retaining systems, which are available from many manufacturers in a wide range of variations, we would like to mention the UNITRAC (Aesculap), which allows any retraction by means of articulated joints and in which a wide range of different blades can be clamped.

In order to operate in the lesser pelvis, holding systems are required which are open cranially and into which a bladder blade can be clamped dorsally (◘ Fig. 3.63).

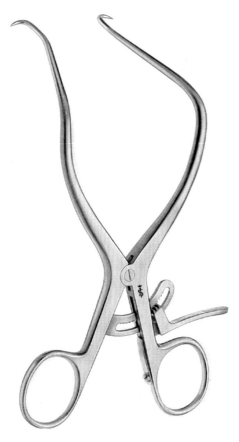

◻ Fig. 3.61 Retractor according to De Bakey. (Aesculap AG, with kind permission)

For the intercostal space, rib retractors have been developed that can be spread slowly by a screw mechanism to prevent rib fracture during spreading (e.g. according to **Finochietto**, ◻ Fig. 3.64). Retractors with fixed blades or with exchangeable blades can be used here.

Alternative thoracic retractors are available according to **Tuffier**, **Haight** or **De Bakey**. The so-called "**Mercedes retractor**" with exchangeable blades is also widely used (◻ Fig. 3.65). There are an infinite number of systems which cannot all be mentioned here. It is important to distinguish whether the frame is fixed to the operating table or can be freely assembled.

3

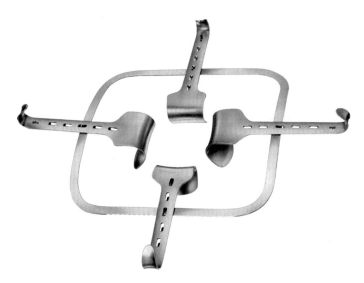

◨ **Fig. 3.62**   Kirschner frame. (Fa. Aesculap AG, with kind permission)

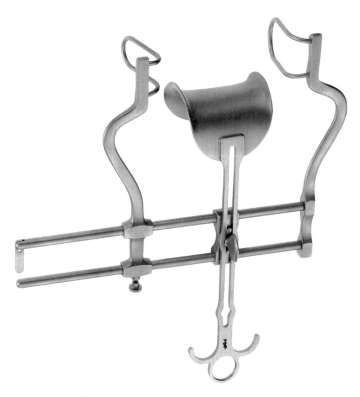

◨ **Fig. 3.63**   Abdominal retractor according to Balfour. (Aesculap AG, with kind permission)

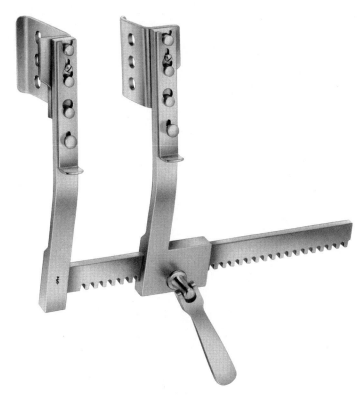

Fig. 3.64 Thoracic retractor according to Finochietto-Burford. (Aesculap AG, with kind permission)

■ Handling

It must be known in advance which frame system is required so that containers do not have to be opened in vain. The systems are often very bulky and therefore difficult to transport.

With all systems, the frame is always attached first, if necessary with the fixation screws for the operating table rails. Then the appropriate blades are used, which are either hooked into the frame or fixed with screw systems. As a rule, the blade is either applied moist or underlaid with a moistened towel to protect the wound tissue.

Self-retaining retractors are grasped by the blades, held horizontally and handed with the blades to open the wound. Each retractor is handed in a closed position.

3

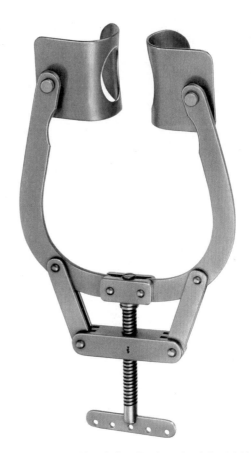

■ **Fig. 3.65**   Mercedes locking device. (Fa. Aesculap AG, with kind permission)

3.1.8 **Needle Holder**

The needle holder resembles a clamp in appearance and construction but is designed **exclusively** to guide a needle.

■ **Shapes**
Length and shape are adapted to the tissue to be sutured. The length and shape of the jaws correspond to this, as do the needle-suture size and shape of the needle. After closing the ratchet, the needle can be locked in the jaws and the surgeon has to open the ratchet every time the tissue layer is penetrated, but there are also needle holders without a catch. These open needle holders are preferably used in dental and maxillofacial surgery. They are available according to **Tönnis** (■ Fig. 3.66) or **Crile**.

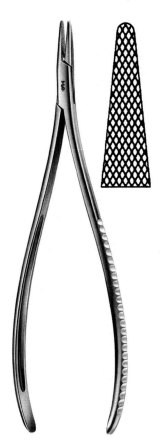

◘ Fig. 3.66 Needle holder according to Tönnis. (Aesculap AG, with kind permission)

Different shapes of handles offer the surgeon the possibility of grasping either in the rings or with the hollow hand around the branches. For example the needle holder according to **Mathieu** (◘ Fig. 3.67), whose branches fit into the hollow hand with their curvature. They have the disadvantage that they require a lot of space and are therefore only suitable for tissue that is easily accessible on the surface.

The long narrower models, e.g. according to **Hegar** (◘ Fig. 3.68), can also be opened and closed easily in the depth of the body. In many cases, these needle holders have a tungsten carbide insert in their jaws to fix the needle. This insert has a grained surface and the needle does not slip or rotate. Again, the gold handle is considered to be the identification of this carbide insert. Alternative names for needle holders include **Crile-Wood**, **Webster**, **Mayo**, **De Bakey**.

3

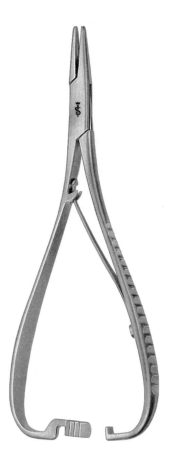

◘ **Fig. 3.67**   Needle holder according to Mathieu. (Aesculap AG, with kind permission)

■ **Mouth Profile**

The grit in the jaws of the needle holders varies in coarseness or fineness so that different sized needles do not destroy the grit. As a result, the nursing staff must select the correct needle holder for the corresponding needle size (◘ Figs. 3.69 and 3.70).

The finest grit is recommended for suture thicknesses 6–0 to 10–0, the medium grit for 4–0 to 6–0, the coarse grit for diameters 3–0 USP and above. Microneedle holders used for needle/thread combinations of 9–0 and above have no profile.

However, carbide inserts with a profile are also gaining ground here (◘ Fig. 3.71).

■ **Handling**

When clamping needles or needle-thread combinations in the needle holder, the size of the needle holder and the grain of the

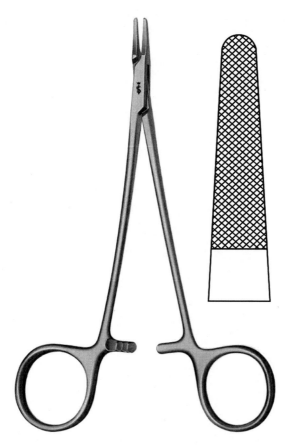

⬛ Fig. 3.68 Needle holder according to Hegar. (Aesculap AG, with kind permission)

jaw profile must be adapted to the size of the needle. The size of the needle also determines how far the ratchet has to be locked.

If a round needle with a thin body planned for intestinal or vascular sutures is clamped in a needle holder with a ratchet, the ratchet only has to lock one grid so that there is a sure grip of the needle but no destruction of the needle by the pressure of the jaws. If a large needle for muscular sutures is clamped in a jaw that is too small, the insert will be destroyed, the needle will have no hold during piercing and the jaws of the needle holder may break under the excessive pressure.

A needle is usually clamped into the needle holder at the range from the posterior third to the middle third of the needle body, so that the right-handed surgeon can see into the needle-rounding and the needle tip points to the left (⬛ Fig. 3.72).

3

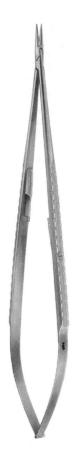

□ **Fig. 3.69**   Needle holder according to Jakobson 1: with ratchet. (Aesculap AG, with kind permission)

For the left-handed operator, the needle tip is clamped pointing to the right (□ Fig. 3.73).

The nurse presents the needle holder to the surgeon in such a way that the curvature of the needle is visible to the surgeon and can be used without delay (□ Fig. 3.74). It must be considered beforehand whether the surgeon is right- or left-handed. Furthermore, it must be considered whether the assisting nurse is standing next to the surgeon or opposite.

The end of the thread is given into the assistant's hand or guided by the assistant until the surgeon ties the first knot. This prevents the thread from becoming entangled and tissue being destroyed by the unintended jerk. The needle holder is grasped at the branch between the needle and the end section and is reached so that the surgeon can reach into the rings.

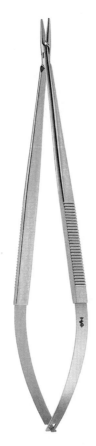

◘ Fig. 3.70   Needle holder according to Jakobson 2: without ratchet. (Aesculap AG, with kind permission)

Some surgeons prefer bent or angled needle holders in poorly accessible areas of the body. The bending of the jaw shows the nurse, how to present the needle-holder. Often the assistant is given an instrument to pull or secure the needle pierced through the tissue. This is usually an empty needle holder, also known as a **needle catcher**.

Many suture manufacturers offer multipacks with the needle attached to the threads in such a way that it can be separated from the thread with a small jerk (tear-off needle, CR = controlled release, Ethicon). However, if this is attempted with an unprepared needle-thread combination, the needle will rotate in the needle holder and wear down the carbide insert or the fixation groove to such an extent that the needles can no longer be held well in position and will rotate when piercing the tissue. A cost-intensive repair is then unavoidable.

3

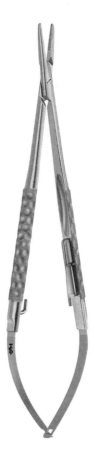

◘ Fig. 3.71   Needle holder according to Castroviejo. (Aesculap AG, with kind permission)

3.1.9 Ligature Needles

In some cases, the **Deschamps** ligation needle is used (◘ Fig. 3.75). It has a simple eye at the tip into which the ligature is threaded. This instrument is available for both right-handers and left-handers; as a rule, the right-handed instrument can be used by all.

The ligature is threaded from the inside to the outside of the eye so that the ligature needle can be removed without unwanted knotting and the ligature comes to lie below the structure. It is then knotted by hand.

The Deschamps is often used in combination with a guiding probe. For this purpose, the probe is pushed under the tissue to be ligated and the hollow channel serves as a guide for the Deschamps. In doing so, it protects the underlying structures (blood vessels, nerves, etc.) from injury. Two Deschamps

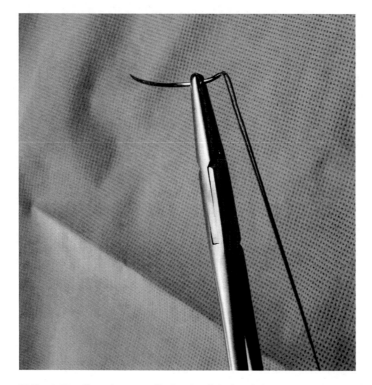

◻ Fig. 3.72 Clamping a needle for the right-handed surgeon. (Photo by Margret Liehn)

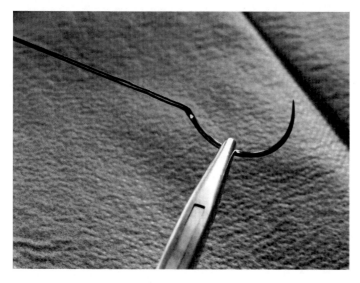

◻ Fig. 3.73 Clamping a needle for the left-handed surgeon. (Photo by Margret Liehn)

3

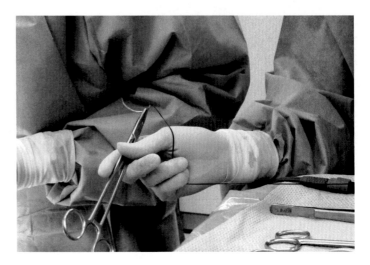

☐ **Fig. 3.74** Presenting a prepared needle holder. (Photo by Margret Liehn)

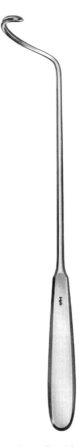

☐ **Fig. 3.75** Deschamps. (Aesculap AG, with kind permission)

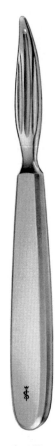

◘ Fig. 3.76 Kocher guiding probe. (Fa. Aesculap AG, with kind permission)

are used to ligate the vessel. After having ligated two-times, the vessel can be cut with dissecting scissors or a scalpel on the lying guiding probe, which also protects the underlying tissue. These guiding probes are available according to **Kocher** (◘ Fig. 3.76), **Kirschner** and **Payr** (◘ Fig. 3.77).

In traumatology, a similar instrument is used to pass steel wire around a bone for a cerclage (▶ Sect. 4.3), this ligation needle is larger to fit the bone.

■ **Handling**

After threading and presenting the guiding probe, which is placed horizontally in the surgeon's hand, the Deschamps is passed diagonally in such a way that the instrument is grasped at the bend under the eye and thus both ligature ends are also grasped so that they do not slip out of the Deschamps on their way to the guiding probe. While the assistant knots the first

3

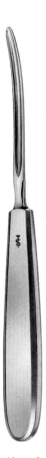

☐ **Fig. 3.77**   Payr guiding probe. (Aesculap AG, with kind permission)

suture, the surgeon receives another ligature threaded into the guiding probe. After both sutures have been placed and knotted, scissors or a scalpel are presented. The tissue is cut in the guide of the probe, then the ligatures are shortened.

Two Deschamps should always be prepared, as threading takes time. The order of presenting and removal may vary, as sometimes one ligation is sufficient. It should be remembered that the body tissue should be cut with a different pair of scissors than is needed to cut the ligatures (▶ Sect. 3.1.3).

Special Instruments

Contents

© Springer-Verlag GmbH Germany, part of Springer Nature 2022
M. Liehn, H. Schlautmann, *101 of Surgical Instruments*, https://doi.org/10.1007/978-3-662-63632-9_4

In addition to the basic instruments that are always required, each surgical department has its own special instruments. The most important ones from various disciplines are presented and explained here. It must always be remembered that a surgeon may have his own preferences, his own ideas about instruments and importance.

Every OR nurse is required to know the instruments used in their unit, to look them up in the instrument catalogue if necessary, and to learn how to handle them.

4.1 Abdominal Surgery

In order to be able to operate in the abdominal cavity, the instruments must correspond in length and shape to the depth of the situs. All the rules that were addressed in the basic instruments chapter also apply here, the designated instruments are identical, but they have a different weight due to the adapted length, which must be considered at the beginning, the handling remains the same.

> Here, too, it is always necessary to consider whether the scrub nurse is standing opposite or next to the surgeon and whether the surgeon is right- or left-handed.

In the following, some special instruments are presented as examples, assigned to the abdominal organs.

4.1.1 Abdomen

After opening the peritoneum, it is obsolete to use sharp instruments that could injure intraperitoneal organs. Thus, sharp retractors are placed on the side table (with the sharp prongs facing upwards or protected by a pad). In many departments, surgical sharp forceps are also put aside, as work usually continues with anatomical or atraumatic forceps (see ► Sect. 3.1.2).

To allow extensive exploration, the assistant doctor lifts the abdominal wall with round retractors and holds it aside so that the surgeon can palpate the situs (◘ Fig. 4.1).

To be able to hold the liver aside atraumatically, so-called liver retractors are used, which are available in various lengths (◘ Fig. 4.2). To protect the organ, a folded, moist towel is placed underneath.

To keep the bowel aside and to protect it, bowel spatulas are used (◘ Fig. 4.3), which are applied moist. Some of these

4

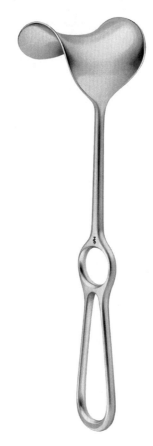

◘ **Fig. 4.1**   Abdominal retractor according to Fritsch. (Aesculap AG, with kind permission)

spatulas are made of flexible material and are manually adapted to the situs. In some cases they have a grooved contact surface to provide support for the retractor.

In the small pelvis, a special angle is needed and firm support for the assistant doctor. For this purpose, a horn is often attached to the handle, which serves as an abutment for the assistant's hand when pulling (◘ Figs. 4.4 and 4.5).

Equivalent retractors exist according to **Deaver**, **Tuffier**, **Doyen** or **Reverdin**, which are not illustrated here.

■   Handling

Retractors are grasped from above and presented horizontally, with the blade facing the patient and the handle facing the surgeon (alternatively the assistant). The retractors can also be grasped at the blade and then presented horizontally.

If retractors remain in the situs for a longer period of time it must be avoided that they stick to the retained organ. To achieve this, they are moistened and, if necessary, a folded

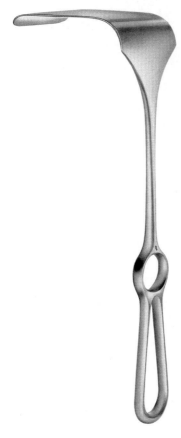

◘ Fig. 4.2 Liver retractor according to Mikulicz. (Aesculap AG, with kind permission)

moist towel is placed between the tissue and the retractor. It is advisable to moisten only the area of the towel that is in contact with the organ.

Hooks are usually prepared in pairs. Intraoperatively, the retractors are changed more frequently in order to be able to take the stage of the operation into account at any time. The used hook is then removed with one hand, while the desired hook is presented with the other hand.

4.1.2 **Esophagus**

In esophageal surgery, it is important to remember that not much traction is applied to the organ so as not further reduce the already low blood flow. As a rule, the esophagus is fastened before dissection. For this purpose, a curved preparation clamp (e.g. according to Overholt, ▶ Chap. 3, ◘ Fig. 3.41) is used to pass under the esophagus and the Overholt is spread.

4

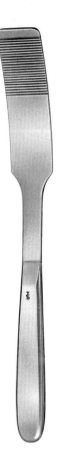

☐ **Fig. 4.3**   Intestinal spatula according to Kader. (Aesculap AG, with kind permission)

A moistened rubber rein is placed between the tips of the mouth and passed below the organ. The two ends of the rubber rein are equipped with a Kocher clamp, so that controlled traction can be exerted on the organ.

If the esophagus is to be detached, an angled clamp is often used, which is applied and, due to its angle, still allows transection without taking up too much space. This clamp must have atraumatic striations because the clamped area is used for the anastomosis. The esophagus must be clamped tightly, as the muscle traction causes the remaining part to contract strongly.

This type of clamp is also used for rectal amputation, which is why it is also called a rectal clamp (☐ Fig. 4.6). It is important to have an angle of approximately 90°, which facilitates the work.

Alternative clamps are those according to **Götze**, **Morris** or **Resano**, which are not shown here.

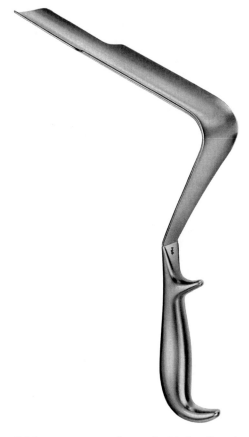

◘ Fig. 4.4 Pelvic retractor according to St. Marks. (Aesculap AG, with kind permission)

■ **Handling**

The clamp is presented closed. It is grasped at its working part and presented with the angle visible. The surgeon grasps the rings and can place the clamp immediately. The organ is then cut, either with a scalpel or a pair of scissors, which is handed to the surgeon immediately after clamping.

4.1.3 **Stomach**

Gastric operations performed openly are becoming less, as both conservative and endoscopic therapies are achieving good results. Nevertheless, some instruments should be mentioned, especially since they are offered with identical jaw shapes in endoscopic therapy.

4

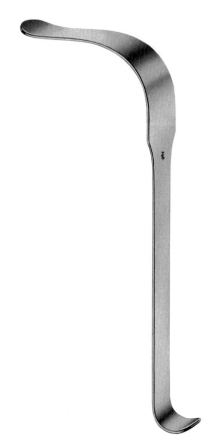

◘ Fig. 4.5   Retractor according to Körte. (Aesculap AG, with kind permission)

Organ clamps (▶ Sect. 3.1.5) are used to clamp the stomach. As the musculature is strongly pronounced, this clamp must be able to grip accordingly. **Babcock**'s tissue forceps have atraumatic striations and are curved in the jaws to provide space for the stomach wall (◘ Fig. 4.7). The tissue forceps according to **Lockwood** can also be used here; due to their light serration, they grasp safe and do not slip off the muscular stomach wall (◘ Fig. 4.8).

Stapling instruments are usually used to remove the stomach (▶ Sect. 4.1.8). However, clamps are also available. It should be borne in mind that a hard clamp is applied to the resectate (e.g. intestinal clamp according to **Hartmann**, ◘ Figs. 4.9 and 4.10) and a soft, atraumatic elastic-closing clamp is applied to the part of the stomach to be anastomosed,

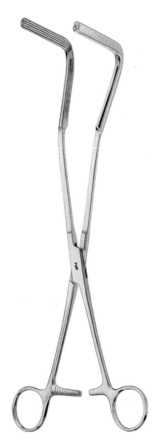

□ **Fig. 4.6** Rectal clamp according to Lloyd-Davis. (Aesculap AG, with kind permission)

which does not destroy the vessels supplying the stomach wall (□ Fig. 4.11).

Comparable clamps are offered according to **Mayo**, **Moynihan** or **Doyen**, they are not shown here.

■ Handling

All instructions given for organ clamps (▶ Sect. 3.1.5) also apply to **Lockwood** or **Babcock** tissue clamps.

During the nursing assistance of a gastric resection, the scrub nurse must recognize which clamp is required, whether a hard or soft elastic clamp must be presented. The clamp is grasped at the jaws and presented in a closed position. The instrument is held diagonally so that the jaws face the stomach when the surgeon grips the rings.

4

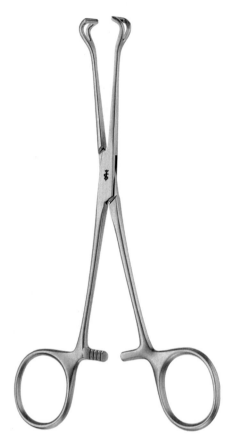

◘ Fig. 4.7   Tissue forceps according to Babcock. (Aesculap AG, with kind permission)

In many cases, holding threads are set at the anastomosis line, which can be further used as corner sutures. These holding threads are placed and equipped with a **Mosquito clamp.** If the thread is to be available as a corner suture, the needle remains on the thread, else it is removed.

Before cutting, the stomach is covered with moist towels to prevent possible contamination of the abdominal cavity with any stomach contents that may escape during cutting. After the clamps have been applied, the stomach is cut. A scalpel can be used here, some surgeons prefer scissors, but the use of a monopolar knife is also possible. When stapling instruments are used, the additional towel covering can be omitted, as the staples close the stomach.

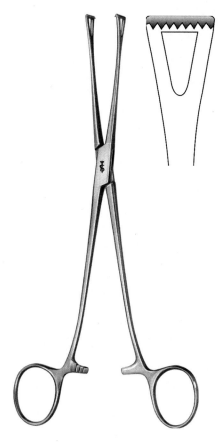

▫ Fig. 4.8 Tissue forceps according to Lockwood. (Aesculap AG, with kind permission)

4.1.4 **Intestine**

The same guidelines as to bowel resections apply as well to gastric resections. The intestinal serosa must be kept moist throughout the operation, for which purpose body-warm moist towels are presented.

Bowel clamps are also available as hard and soft elastic clamps, whereby it should be noted that hard clamps are applied to the resected part and soft, elastic clamps are required on the part to be anastomosed in order to ensure a sufficient blood supply to the anastomosis. The bowel is cut between the clamps with a scalpel or scissors. Moist abdomi-

4

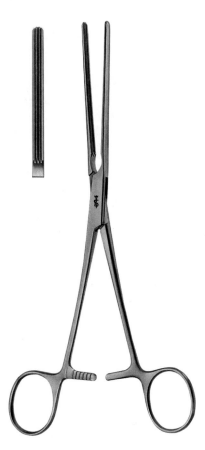

◘ Fig. 4.9 Intestinal clamp according to Hartmann. (Aesculap AG, with kind permission)

nal towels are placed around the bowel to protect the surrounding tissues from contamination in case of leakage of bowel contents.

In addition to the bowel clamps according to **Kocher** or **Hartmann** (◘ Figs. 4.9 and 4.10), the **Satinsky clamp**, ▸ Chap. 3, ◘ Fig. 3.40) or 90° clamps are used here, too. The soft elastic bowel clamps (e.g. according to **Kocher**) are often additionally covered with a tube gauze to protect the serosa. In this case it is necessary to moisten the clamps before use!

Since in the context of **fast-track surgery** or in emergency surgery the patient's bowel is not always cleaned by ortho- and/or retrograde irrigation, many surgeons feel is advantageous to clean the ends of the bowel after resection and before anastomosis with a swab soaked in disinfectant. Under no circumstances is an alcoholic solution used here, but as a rule a disinfectant containing iodine.

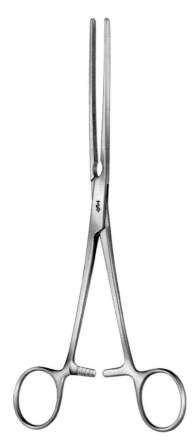

◻ Fig. 4.10 Bowel clamp according to Kocher. (Aesculap AG, with kind permission)

In rectal surgery, it must be considered that the possibilities of instrument movement are limited in the small pelvis and therefore very long retractor systems and, if necessary, also long dissecting instruments must be kept in standby, sometimes with multiple bends in the branches. In order to be able to dissect without problems, the scissors (◻ Fig. 4.12) and also the needle holder (◻ Fig. 4.13) are strongly bent in the jaws or also in the handle, if necessary, or they have an additional joint.

▪ Handling

All the criteria already mentioned apply to the use of the bowel clamps. The scrub nurse knows the procedure, the names of the instruments and the sequence of the material to be applied. In case of doubt, the instruments are moistened before use.

4

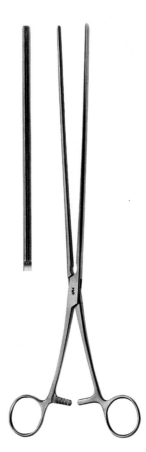

◘ **Fig. 4.11**   Gastric clamp according to Scudder. (Aesculap AG, with kind permission)

In the case of an additionally bent jaw or S-shaped handle, the bend of the jaw must follow the shape of the organ during use. To protect the moist mucous membranes, body-warm rinsing solution is kept ready.

4.1.5 **Spleen**

Removal of the spleen is only an option if all other therapeutic options have failed or if spleen preservation is not possible in the case of trauma. In such cases, clamps are needed for the splenic hilum which, because of their curvature, do not obstruct the view of the situs, e.g. the **Satinsky clamp** (▶ Chap. 3, ◘ Fig. 3.40). It should be borne in mind that the organ bleeds very profusely when injured, so that instrument presen-

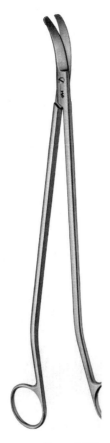

◘ Fig. 4.12 Rectal scissors according to Müller, S-shaped. (Aesculap AG, with kind permission)

tation must proceed rapidly and the suction device must be functional.

If the organ is preserved despite rupture and bleeding, haemostatic options must be kept ready, such as non-contact coagulation, haemostatic tissue, meshes made of absorbable or partially absorbable material and/or the option of infrared coagulation. Here, the internal OR standards should be consulted before preparation.

4.1.6 **Liver/Biliary**

Removal of the gallbladder is performed using a minimally invasive approach (▶ Sect. 4.2). In rare cases, it is necessary to convert to the conventional method, in which case special instruments must be prepared.

4

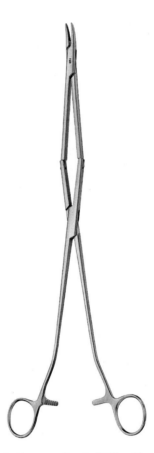

◘ Fig. 4.13   Needle holder according to Müller. (Aesculap AG, with kind permission)

In addition to the liver retractors and, if necessary, intestinal spatula (◘ Fig. 4.3), gallbladder grasping forceps (► Chap. 3, ◘ Fig. 3.46), dissecting scissors and longer anatomical tissue forceps and ligature clamps according to **Overholt** must be kept at hand. If the choledochal duct has to be revised, a stab scalpel is required and angled scissors (e.g. according to **Potts de Martell**, ► Chap. 3, ◘ Fig. 3.27) to widen the stab incision.

There are various options for removing stones that may be present in the bile duct. Stones can be removed via a Fogarty catheter, but bendable spoons (according to **Körte**) or stone grasping forceps can also be helpful (◘ Fig. 4.14). These have no ratchet so that stones of different calibres can be grasped and removed from the duct.

Instruments for dilating the papilla Vateri (dilators) or for placing a T-drainage into the choledochal duct (T-drainage, straight scissors, thin suture material) are only used very rarely.

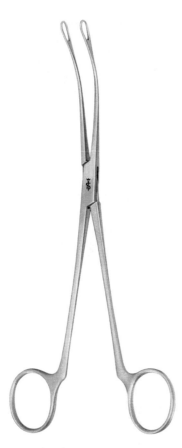

☐ **Fig. 4.14** Stone grasping forceps according to Blake. (Aesculap AG, with kind permission)

An operation on the liver in visceral surgery is usually based on a tumour or a traumatic event with rupture and bleeding.

As a result, in addition to the basic instruments (▶ Sect. 3.1.4), retractors and self-retaining systems must be provided which correspond to the length of the patient's body. Since major bleeding is to be expected in the event of trauma, sufficient towels and body-warm irrigation solution must be kept ready. Staplers are usually used for a partial resection (▶ Sect. 4.1.8). In case of trauma a cell-saving system is used as a suction device so that the aspirated blood can be re-infused into the patient.

▪ **Handling**

The rules already discussed apply to all of the above instruments. The scrub nurse knows the indication and can prepare the instruments accordingly in a standardized manner. In case

4

of traumatic ruptures, at least one suction must be kept ready, as well as sufficient towels and irrigation fluid. Sometimes haemostasis is achieved temporarily via "packing", in which case warm moist towels are placed on the rupture for approximately 24 hours to achieve haemostasis by compression. Attention must be paid to the correct documentation of the number of the textile towels **intentionally** remaining in the patient.

Coagulation, mono- or bipolar, as well as non-contact argon coagulation is possible, furthermore an absorbable mesh can be applied for compression. If necessary, a tourniquet is applied over the hepatoduodenal ligament in order to specifically restrict the blood supply (Pringle maneuver). For this purpose, a strong band is passed around the ligament, a short (1–1.5 cm) rubber tube is pulled over both ends of the band and a clamp is applied over it to hold the rubber tube in position. Depending on the requirements, a compression of the vessel can be achieved and the blood supply can be specifically reduced. A **Satinsky clamp** can also be used for the Pringle maneuver.

4.1.7 Pancreas

Basic and laparotomy instruments are required for interventions on the pancreas. It should be borne in mind that pancreatic juice is aggressive, so the surrounding tissue must be protected with moist towel drapes. If resection is planned, stapling instruments can be used.

4.1.8 Stapler

The use of stapling suture instruments has become indispensable in abdominal surgery, as stapled sutures have many advantages and the recovering of patients, e.g. after bowel resections, is shortened. The pressure of the single clamp of the Stapler on the intestinal tissue as well as the blood supply of the organ is constantly reliable. The anastomoses created with a Stapler are considered gas- and water- proof.

Most companies offer the staplers as disposable instruments. There are different types of instruments whose staple-magazines can be reloaded as required. Depending on the field of application, 30, 60 or 90 mm long magazines are used. The staples are made of titanium or of resorbable material. In the magazine the staples have an U-shape and after releasing the stapling mechanism they are formed into a lying "B". This shape secures blood flow to the intestinal walls. Almost all stapler models are also manufactured for endoscopic use.

Currently, three types of devices are distinguished:
- **Linear Stapler** (■ Fig. 4.15)
  - Linear (linea: line) means straight. A linear stapling instrument places staples in a straight line and thus closes a hollow organ. The shaft of the instrument can be straight, curved or angled, the working part, in which the staple magazine is located, is straight and places at least two or more rows of staples in parallel, which seal the tissue air- and waterproof.
- **Linear Cutter** (■ Fig. 4.16)
  - These instruments are used to close and simultaneously cut through of the bowel. This allows the creation of a side-to-side anastomosis. The instrument first clamps with at least two parallel rows of clamps and then cuts through the tissue with an integrated knife.
  - The staples are between 50 and 100 mm long, depending on the application, and the staple length is selected between 2.5–4.8 mm, depending on the tissue to be stapled.

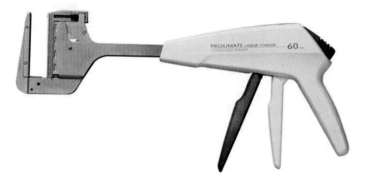

■ **Fig. 4.15** Linear Stapler TX60. (Ethicon, with kind permission)

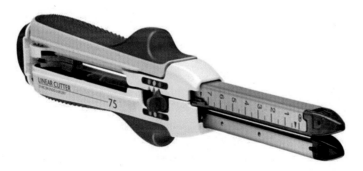

■ **Fig. 4.16** Linear Cutter NTLC -01. (Ethicon, by courtesy)

4

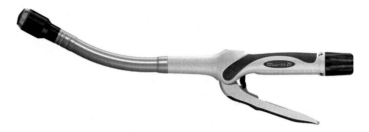

◘ Fig. 4.17 Circular Stapler CDH29A.1. (Ethicon, with kind permission)

— **Circular Stapler (◘** Fig. 4.17)
  – These instruments are used to create an end-to-end anastomosis by clamping two lumina with 4 staple-lines and cutting between the lines with an integrated knife. Two lines stay at the organ, two lines are excised. These excised lines must be examined for completeness and integrity in order to evaluate the quality of the anastomosis. At the same time, these lines can be examined histologically to provide information whether the resection margins are tumor-free.
  – The fact that the instrument head is removable makes it easier to create anastomoses intraoperatively, e.g. a very deep rectal anastomosis can be created by knotting the instrument head in the sigmoid and inserting the stapler via the anus. The instrument shaft is curved or straight to varying degrees. The curved ones are easier to insert and ensure a better view. The size of the instrument head determines the diameter of the anastomosis (21–33 mm), the staples all have a length of 5.5 mm.
  – With the different instruments offered, the closing pressure of the clamps can sometimes be regulated manually, so that the shape of the lying "B" can vary and the tissue trauma can be controlled individually.
  – For the creation of an anastomosis with the circular stapler, purse string sutures are required which allow the instrument head to be tied in. By applying a purse string clamp (◘ Fig. 4.18), the correct application of this suture is possible.

■ **Handling**
Each OR nurse knows the stapling instruments used in the OR unit and the magazines kept at hand. It is important to make the instruments ready for use before presenting them and, if necessary, loading the instrument with the desired staple magazine. Since the instruments are often only provided by the cir-

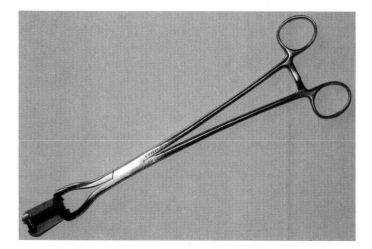

◘ Fig. 4.18 Purse string clamp. (Ethicon, with kind permission)

culating nurse directly before use, in order to avoid unnecessary opening of the expensive instruments, the preparation must be quick and accordingly known.

After preparation and insertion of the desired magazine, the staples are grasped at the magazine and handed with the handle in a way that the surgeon can grasp the release handles and the instrument head points to the surgical area. If anal anastomosis is planned, lubricating gel, intestinal tube and, if required, dyed irrigation solution should be ready.

4.2 MIS Instruments

Operations with minimally invasive access are to be expected in every surgical discipline. The technical equipment is usually available on a video trolley (◘ Fig. 4.19); every member of staff in the operating theatre is familiar with the equipment, its mode of operation and its most frequent sources of error. The operation is observed by the entire team on one or better several monitors, the positioning of these monitors must meet the ergonomic requirements of the entire team. Every employee has been instructed to operate these technical devices and to be able to correctly connect all tubes and cables to the tower.

Access to the target organ is provided via trocars, and daylight-like conditions are created by an optical system connected to a cold light source. In order to obtain space in the intraperitoneal cavity, prewarmed carbon dioxide (CO_2) is insufflated, which inflates the abdominal cavity and thus cre-

4

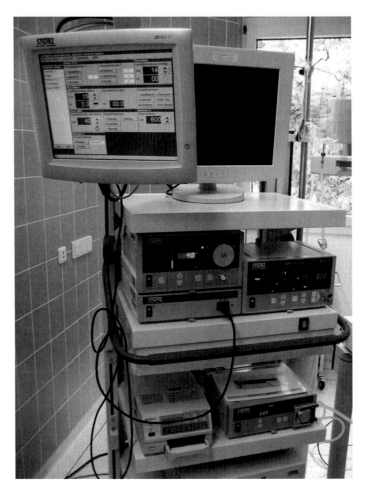

Fig. 4.19 Laparoscopic tower. (From: Carus (2014)

ates open space. Insufflation devices indicate the pressure that exists in the intraperitoneal space, as well as the volume that is being infused. The insufflation speed is adjusted via the "flow"-dial on the insufflator.

4.2.1 **Trocars**

The trocar provides access to the surgical site. Instruments and optics are navigated in place via it. They are available as disposable as well as reusable instruments. They have a **stylet** or **obturator** that fills the interior of the instrument during insertion (■ Fig. 4.20). Mandrins come pointed and blunt. Pointed in order to be able to perforate the tissue layers, blunt if access to the intraperitoneal cavity has already been created via a

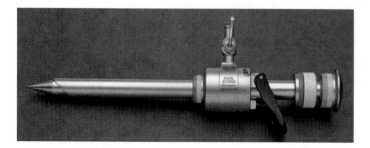

■ **Fig. 4.20**   10 mm trocar and obturator. (From: Carus (2014))

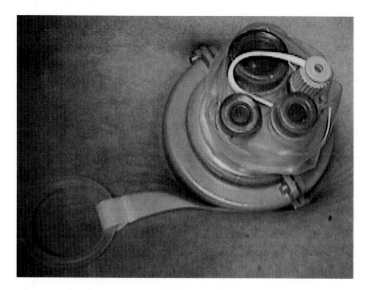

■ **Fig. 4.21**   Example of a single port. (From: Carus (2014))

small incision. The obturator is removed after placement of the trocar, thus creating space for the needed instrument.

Either two to five trocars are used or a "single port" positioned at the umbilicus is inserted (■ Fig. 4.21), through which instruments and optics (usually three ports) can be put in place. The diameter of the trocars must correspond to the required instruments (5 mm, 10 mm, 12 mm), offer the possibility of insufflation or enable the using of smaller calibre instruments without gas loss by means of adaptors.

Frequently, the first trocar is placed in the intraperitoneal space via a small incision under visualization using a semi-open technique, and gas insufflation is performed via this incision. These trocars have a rounded tip (**Hasson trocar**) to avoid injury to organs. For the treatment of an inguinal hernia, for example, there are trocars with a balloon; tissue dissection can be performed via the air-filled balloon.

4

4.2.2 **Optics**

The optics consist of the funnel-shaped eyepiece with connection for the camera system, the connection for the cold light conducting cable and the shaft in which the lens system is housed (◘ Fig. 4.22). The shaft diameter should be as small as possible, mostly this is possible with a rod lens system, the so-called **Hopkins optics**. Depending on the application, the diameter is 2–3 mm (in pediatric surgery), 5 mm and 10 mm.

Sometimes bendable tips are needed, but this reduces the viewing conditions. The direction of view provided by the optic is given in degrees. The 0° straight-ahead optic allows a direct view of an organ, but it cannot be rotated. 30°, 70° and 90° optics are so-called angle optics. They allow a view of structures that cannot be seen via direct view, which is why they are usually preferred.

In many cases, the optics contain a CCD chip in the distal end of the optics, which allows the image to be transmitted digitally to the monitor. The fiber optic cable that is connected to the optics should be long enough to ensure the distance between the non-sterile and sterile areas.

The diameter of the cable contributes significantly to the quality of the image on the monitor and should be 5 mm in diameter for a 10 mm optic (◘ Figs. 4.23 and 4.24). The camera is a mountable chip camera that provides detailed color-correct images. The camera system is linked to the possibility of digital recording via a video recorder or a video printer for documentation.

■ Handling

The instruments required in MIS correspond in their jaws to those known from conventional surgery. However, as the path leads through the trocars to the target organ, they must be longer; the jaws can often be turned by means of a dial on the handle. The instruments are available as disposable and reusable instruments.

MIS instruments are hollow-shaft instruments approximately 30 cm long; reusable instruments must be able to be disassembled for reprocessing. Here, too, there are grasping forceps, scissors, dissection instruments, clamps, needle holders and HF electrodes for mono- or bipolar coagulation, corresponding to those known from conventional surgery.

Grasping clamps are used instead of forceps. The same rules apply to the shape of the jaws and their teeth as have already been mentioned for conventional instruments. The clamps should grip, and the extent to which the tissue may be

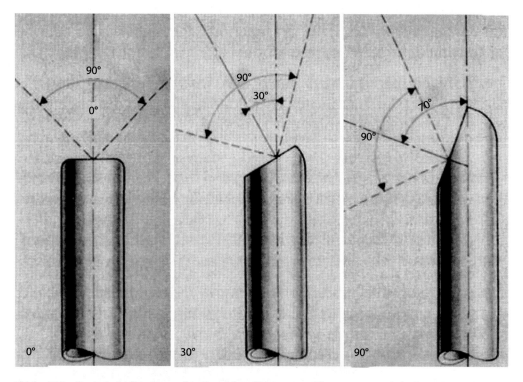

Fig. 4.22 Typical viewing planes of optics with rod lens system. The aperture angle is always 90°, while there are options with a viewing plane of 0°, 30° and 70°, for example. Different angles are chosen depending on the indication. (From Wintermantel and Suk-Woo (2009))

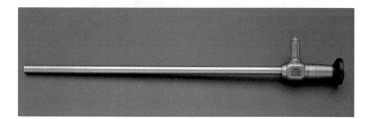

Fig. 4.23 10-mm optic. (From: Carus (2014))

traumatized or crushed must be considered. The jaw shape is selected accordingly (**□** Figs. 4.25, 4.26, and 4.27).

Organ forceps have a jaw approximately 30 mm long with transverse serrations to allow grasping and clamping of the intra-abdominal organs. A dial near the handle allows free rotation through 360° in both directions. The handle is usually lockable so that they can be used as holding forceps.

4

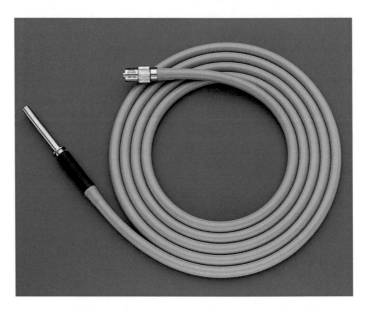

Fig. 4.24 Fibre optic cable. (From: Carus (2014))

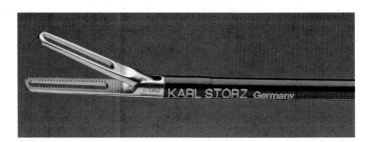

Fig. 4.25 Grasping forceps for minimally invasive surgery 1. (From: Carus (2014))

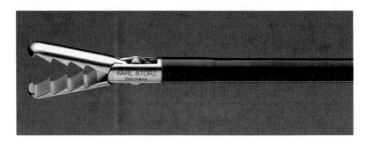

Fig. 4.26 Grasping forceps for minimally invasive surgery 2. (From: Carus (2014))

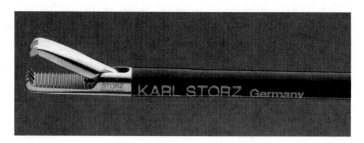

▣ Fig. 4.27 Grasping forceps for minimally invasive surgery 3. (From: Carus (2014))

The coarser the tissue, the stronger the forceps selected must be. The naming of the forceps is either based on their purpose (lung grasping forceps) or is chosen analogously to the conventional instrument (e.g. **Babcock forceps**). Sometimes the names also show the associations made by the shape of the jaws (crocodile forceps). For dissection, the Overholt is also applied here.

Since in minimally invasive surgery the preparation is often blunt, some forceps are supplied with an attachment for the coagulation cable, then the spread tissue can be coagulated and cut simultaneously.

Retractors are used for holding and lifting tissue. (▣ Fig. 4.28). They can be deployed in the intraperitoneal space after insertion via the trocar.

A special hook can be used as a retractor, but with a connection for high frequency or ultrasound it can also be used for dissection (▣ Fig. 4.29). By applying monopolar current, tissue can be coagulated and severed with the hook bent at about 90° at the tip.

The scissors also correspond to those already known, the **Metzenbaum** scissors are most frequently used, but scissors with one hook are also used, which can take up tissue on a blade by means of the hook shape and thus cut selectively (▣ Figs. 4.30 and 4.31).

If suturing is required, two needle holders are used, as both ends of the thread must be grasped to form the knot if intracorporeal knotting is to be performed. Instead of the intracorporeal knot, the knot can also be preformed extracorporeally, which is then brought to the knot point with a knot pusher.

As suturing and knotting in minimally invasive surgery takes time and the learning curve is relatively flat, clips are often preferred (▣ Fig. 4.32). Titanium clips are inserted using an applicator, placed over the structure to be closed and

4

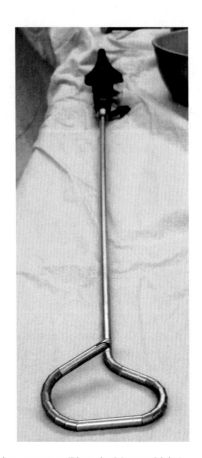

Fig. 4.28 Liver retractor. (Photo by Margret Liehn)

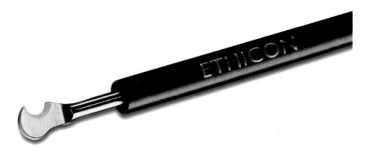

Fig. 4.29 Tactile hook for ultrasound preparation. (From: Carus (2014))

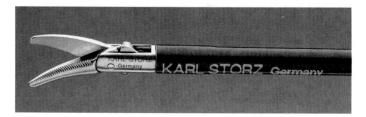

◼ **Fig. 4.30** Scissors for minimally invasive surgery 1. (From: Carus (2014))

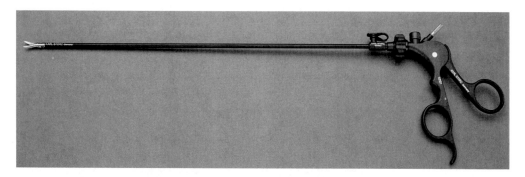

◼ **Fig. 4.31** Scissors for minimally invasive surgery 2. (From: Carus (2014))

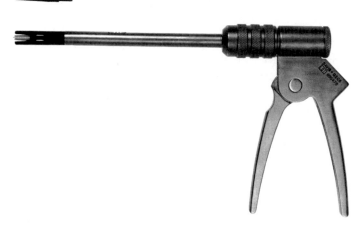

◼ **Fig. 4.32** Example of a clip applicator in minimally invasive surgery. (From: Carus (2014))

4

closed with the handle of the instrument. The free end of the clip closes first so that no tissue can escape. Between the applied clips, the tissue is cut with scissors. Instead of titanium, resorbable material (polydioxanone) can be used.

It is important to remember that different clips have their own applicator, otherwise the clips will get lost on their way through the trocar.

■ **Handling**

Instrumentation in minimally invasive surgery follows different criteria than that in "conventional" surgery. The view of the monitor must be possible, and in the case of conversion to an "open" procedure, the required instruments must be able to be prepared quickly and in a standardized manner.

Reusable MIS instruments have to be sterilized in disassembled form and assembled preoperatively in the operating room by the scrub nurse. This process must be practiced in a non-sterile state in order to avoid time delays. Even if the instrument set is assembled and sterilized in the container trays from the CSSD, there are many work steps:

— The trocars are assembled, the valves or flaps closed, rubber seals fitted if necessary, the obturator inserted.
— Threads must be loosely tightened, as it is not allowed to be closed for steam sterilization.
— Instruments with insulated shafts for high-frequency surgery are checked for damage; if such damage is detected, they must be replaced.
— Liquids on the table are marked with a code that is valid for the entire department so that, for example, rinsing solution and anti-fogging agent cannot be confused.
— Clip applicators are filled with the required clips, each clip shape has its specific applicator, usually only one clip can be clamped.

Due to the shape and application of the instruments, the presentation is different. On the one hand, the instruments are very delicate and long, so that care must be taken to grasp the centre of the instrument so the instrument is not bent while it is being presented. Some surgeons prefer the insertion of the instrument with help to the trocar shaft so that they not have to look away from the monitor.

In the operating room it is darkened because the ceiling light is not needed. Often forceps and scissors look very similar externally and can only be distinguished on closer inspection.

Therefore each instrument has its own fixed place on the instrument table, so that there is no risk of confusion.

The shaft of the instruments must be cleaned after use because blood adhesions increase resistance when repeatedly inserted into the trocar shaft. Hollow-shaft instruments are rinsed intraoperatively to prevent protein build-up, to facilitate reprocessing. It should be borne in mind that physiological saline solution corrodes instruments (▶ Sect. 7.2.1). Aqua destillata, for example, is suitable for flushing.

The OR staff knows the order of application of the desired **trocars**. The valves of the trocars are closed (they are opened for sterilization), the correct obturator is inserted. The trocar is grasped by the tip and held vertically and presented to the surgeon after the skin incision is made with a scalpel. After positioning, the obturator is removed, taken by the scrub nurse, and the following instrument, starting with the optic, is presented briskly to avoid gas loss. When using single ports, the preparation of the model used must be known.

The **optics** are mostly autoclaved in sterile condition incl. Camera system and can be used without a sterile cover. If this is not the case, the optics are covered with a sterile transparent tube system. The scrub nurse holds the optics to which was fixed the sterile tubular film (with the adhesive strip integrated in the tubular film), the circulating nurse connects the camera to the eyepiece and then pulls the turned over tubular film far into the non-sterile area.

The optics fog up due to the different temperatures outside and inside the abdominal cavity. To fight fog, industrially manufactured solution can be applied to the glass surface with a swab. Intraoperatively, this may become necessary if the optic becomes "blind" due to the application of high-frequency current or ultrasound dissection. The optic with the desired angle is grasped at the shaft and presented diagonally to the surgeon, who immediately inserts it into the prepared trocar.

Graspers, grasping forceps, scissors and **swab forceps** usually have the same shape. The scrub nurse knows into which trocar the requested instrument is to be inserted and must prepare an adaptor if necessary. These instruments are grasped in the middle of the long shaft and handed at an angle with the tip pointing towards the trocar, so that the surgeon can grasp the rings of the instrument and insert it promptly into the trocar.

Rod retractors are used when the use of gravity alone is not sufficient to hold organs aside. To hold a liver lobe out of the field of view, a rod is sometimes sufficient, but a self-retaining retractor may also be used. The nurse presents the retractor in a folded state and the surgeon opens the instrument in situ.

Needle holders are prepared in pairs, as two instruments are needed to tie the knot. Some skilled surgeons take an Overholt as a second instrument. The required threads are

4

shortened to a predetermined length and the needle is clamped in such a way that the needle holder with needle can be measured in place through the working trocar, the second needle holder is passed over another trocar for knotting.

Knot sliders are needed when the surgeon has knotted the suture outside the abdominal cavity (extracorporeally) and the knot needs to be guided to the situs. **Clip applicators** must fit the required clips. To fit the clip into the instrument, the applicator must be placed on the loading unit at a predetermined angle. When presenting, the handles must not be touched to avoid involuntary squeezing which would cause the clip to fall out.

The handling of the absorbable clips is more difficult. They too must be inserted absolutely correctly into the application forceps, but before insertion the forceps must be half closed, as with the clip fully open the diameter of the trocar is insufficient for insertion.

With some manufacturers it is necessary to fix the clip in the correct position with the fingertip after loading the applicator.

4.3 Instruments Used in Traumatology and Orthopaedics Department

In traumatology, the basic instruments required are identical to those in abdominal surgery, but much smaller in quantity. In this chapter, **only** basic bone instruments will be discussed, since implants and osteosynthesis systems are so different and varied that it would go beyond the scope of this book. Reference can only be made here to surgical textbooks and manufacturers' manuals.

4.3.1 Raspatories

After cutting through the soft tissue, the periosteum is detached from the bone with the raspatory (Latin: raspare: to rasp) to such an extent that the cortical bone is exposed where, for example, the fracture lies or is to be sawn. Adhering soft tissue is scraped off with this instrument in order to be able to perform an osteosynthesis. To do this, this instrument must fit firmly in the surgeon's hand and be sharply ground so that it can scrape off the periosteum but not roughen the cortex.

A raspatory consists of the handle, a shaft and ends in the working part, also called the "blade" (◻ Figs. 4.33, 4.34, and 4.35). This blade can be rectangular or rounded, either the

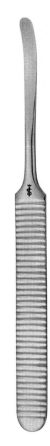

◘ **Fig. 4.33** Raspatory according to Williger. (Aesculap AG, with kind permission)

sides are also sharpened or only the rounded working end is sharp. The handle is grooved to give a firm grip or has a groove to hold the index finger during the working process.

To test whether the working end is sharpened, you can run your fingertip over the working end. A sharp edge can be felt (compare this to a dissector, which may look similar from a distance, but has a blunt working end!). There are instruments with two working ends, one side sharp like a raspatory, one side blunt like a dissector.

Here, special attention is required for handling.

Comparable raspatories according to **Adson**, **Cottle**, **Joseph** or **König** are not shown here. Double-ended raspatories are also used, in which case one end is often straight and the other bent.

If the instruments are split at the blade, so-called dovetail raspatories, they are used on bone edges; if they are strongly bent, they are popular on the jawbone. For the removal of the periosteum at the rib, special shapes are necessary in order to

4

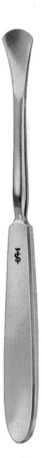

◻ **Fig. 4.34**   Raspatory according to Langenbeck. (Aesculap AG, with kind permission)

protect the pleura and still be able to scrape effectively (◻ Fig. 4.36). For this purpose, the end of the shaft is ring-shaped but open so that it can be placed around the rib and the periosteum of the back of the rib can also be loosened. This instrument is available open to the right or to the left so that it can be used for both hands.

Today, many raspatories are offered with plastic handles, different colours can be chosen to distinguish them.

▪ **Handling**

The nurse grasps the raspatory by its working part, held at a slight angle and the surgeon grasps the handle. The ground end points towards the bone (◻ Fig. 4.37).

Double-sided instruments are grasped at the part of the instrument required by the surgeon. If the instrument is curved, the bending follows the bone edge during the approach.

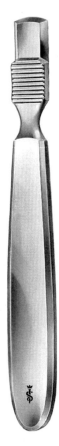

Fig. 4.35 Raspatory according to Farabeuf. (Aesculap AG, with kind permission)

4.3.2 Periostal Elevator and Bone Lever

The name of this instrument also comes from the Latin language (elevare: to lift up). This blunt instrument can be used to lift bone fragments or small bones in order to carry out a reduction or to lift an impressed bone (e.g. on the skull bone). The elevator has a handle, a shaft and a working part, but in contrast to the raspatory, the latter is round - i.e. bluntly ground (☐ Fig. 4.38).

As already described, there is an instrument according to **Freer** which is double-ended, sharp on one side like a raspatory, blunt on the other side like an elevator or a dissector.

Caution and attention to presentation is required here.

Comparable elevators - not shown - are named after **Langenbeck** or **Williger.**

4

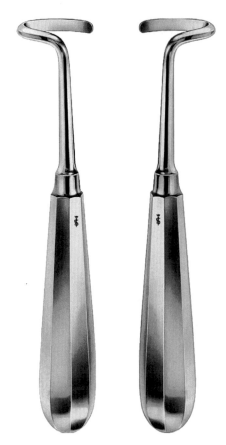

◻ Fig. 4.36 Rib raspatory according to Doyen. (Aesculap AG, with kind permission)

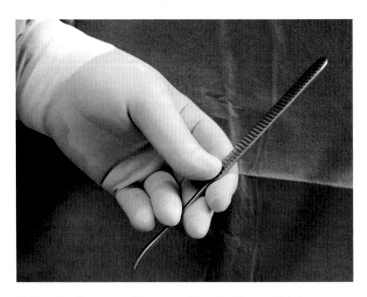

◻ Fig. 4.37 Presenting a Raspatory. (Photo by Margret Liehn)

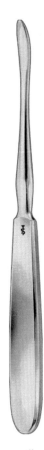

◘ Fig. 4.38 Periostal elevator according to Quervain. (Fa. Aesculap AG, with kind permission)

The term "bone lever" is not common, but the "**Hohmann lever**" is the best known of the bone levers. These are relatively strong instruments, consisting of a curved handle ending in a broad blade, which has a rounded curved tip in the middle (◘ Fig. 4.39).

The tip and the blade are pushed under the bone to be lifted and with the strong handle the bone can be lifted and/or the muscles can be held away from the bone in order to be able to saw, for example, at the femoral head. This instrument is also available in many variations, the use is identical.

The size of the instrument depends on the surgical area; at the hip, the lever is much longer and wider than at the wrist or ankle. Comparable bone levers - not shown here - are available, for example, according to **Verbrugge**.

■ Handling

The presentation of an elevator is identical to that described for the raspatory (◘ Fig. 4.37). The bone lever is grasped at

4

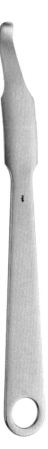

◨ **Fig. 4.39** Bone lever according to Hohmann. (Aesculap AG, with kind permission)

the upwardly curved tip and is given diagonally so that it can be brought in place at the planned site without having to be rotated (◨ Fig. 4.40). In standardized operations, it is usually described which lever is required when and in which position.

4.3.3 Bone Retractor with One Sharp Prong

To lift bone fragments, sharp single prong retractors are available in many sizes (◨ Fig. 4.41).

Comparable retractors are named after **Volkmann.** The handling and presenting corresponds to that discussed for the sharp hooks (► Sect. 3.1.6).

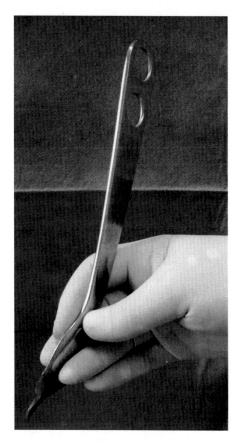

Fig. 4.40 Presenting a bone lever according by Hohmann. (Photo by Margret Liehn)

4.3.4 **Bone Curettes**

In order to be able to remove impacted bone parts or periosteum remnants from the fracture gap, an instrument is used that comes from dentistry. It has a special shape and a working part on both sides. They are named after **Lucas** or **Hemingway** (■ Fig. 4.42).

There are curettes for the same function, they exist in many forms, straight, bent in the working part, angled and with different sized curettes. They are named after **Volkmann** (■ Fig. 4.43), **Schede** and others.

■ Handling

The scrub nurse knows (or asks for) the desired tray size and whether the material being scraped should be retained. The

4

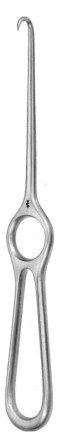

❑ **Fig. 4.41**   Bone retractor according to Kocher. (Aesculap AG, with kind permission)

instrument is grasped by the working part, held at a slight angle and the surgeon grasps the handle so that the working surface points to the bone. If the material is to be stored or given for histological examination, a small bowl is ready, if necessary filled with NaCl solution or covered with a moist towel.

4.3.5 Chisel and Hammer

Chisels are sharp instruments that have a handle and a sharply ground blade at the working end. They are needed to cut through bone or split off a part. Flat shaped chisels used to split off parts of bone are often called **osteotomes**. The blade can be straight, which is the so-called **flat chisel**, or hollow shaped as in the so-called **gouge**.

The grind of the blade varies, may be ground on both sides or one side, bent or straight shaped, or have a split point for

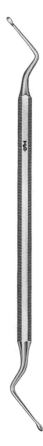

☐ **Fig. 4.42** Bone curette according to Hemingway. (Aesculap AG, with kind permission)

special use. As a rule, they have a strong rectangularly shaped handle made of plastic so that the hammer has a large contact surface (☐ Fig. 4.44). An exception to this is the **Lambotte** chisel (often called an osteotome), which is made entirely of metal. The blade is ground on both sides (☐ Fig. 4.45).

The size of the chisel is adapted to the bone to be separated. The handle can also be bayonet-shaped in order to be used on the septum in otorhinolaryngology, for example. The chisel according to **Lebsche**, which is rarely used, has a special shape (☐ Fig. 4.46). It was designed to cut through the sternum, for which purpose it has a right-angled bent tip, the blade of which is ground on one side; the right angle is used as a "shoe" to protect the soft tissues. The cane-like handle allows a firm grip and good guidance on the sternum.

The chisel known as Tamper with a blunt, cross-grooved working end is used to insert and compact cancellous bone chips (☐ Fig. 4.47). In the catalogues, it is often still considered a "haemostatic chisel".

4

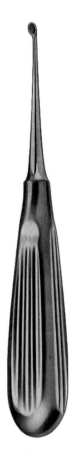

◘ Fig. 4.43 Bone curette according to Volkmann. (Aesculap AG, with kind permission)

A hammer is needed to drive the sharp chisel into the bone with force. The hammers are either metal or plastic, the rule being that a plastic handle may only be struck with a plastic hammer, while a metal chisel must be driven in with a metal hammer. A metal hammer could cause cracks in the plastic handle, which could make proper reprocessing difficult or impossible. The hammer consists of a handle and the hammer head, which is used to strike the chisel.

■ **Handling**

Chisels are grasped at the working end and held vertically before being given to the surgeon's **left** hand. Gouges point with the hollow side towards the bone cutting edge. Following the presenting of the chisel, the surgeon immediately receives the hammer (corresponding to the handle of the chisel) in the **right** hand. To do this, the nurse grasps the hammer head,

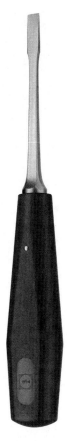

◘ Fig. 4.44 Chisel according to Lexer. (Aesculap AG, with kind permission)

holds the instrument horizontally and then gives the handle to the surgeon (◘ Fig. 4.48).

If bone is removed with the hammer and chisel, again, a small bowl must be prepared to hold bone chips or bone blocks until they are needed.

In this regard, it should be noted that extracted material should always be transported only above the sterile tables, so that if it slips out of the nurses or the surgeon's hand, it does not fall on the floor under any circumstances.

4.3.6 Bone Forceps, Reposition Forceps

In some cases, the bone must be held, the repositioning temporarily be fixed or part of the bone removed with gouge forceps. The bone forceps usually do not have rings that the surgeon

4

◘ Fig. 4.45   Chisel according to Lambotte. (Aesculap AG, with kind permission)

grips into, but instead have branches that are grooved on the outside to prevent the hand from slipping off.

Since bones have a hard structure, these instruments must be adapted to the force and size of the bone. These forceps have a jaw shaped according to the task, a closing mechanism usually offered without locking, sometimes with a double transmission so as not to take up too much space in the situs and two branches.

Some forceps can be fixed in their holding function by a screw lock (forceps according to **Ulrich**). Bone holding forceps have a toothed jaw to grip and hold the bone, but not to cut or injure it. They are offered straight, bent, and bent sideways. Some of these forceps are also named after their appearance, e.g. the "**lion's mouth**", which is actually named as bone holding forceps after **Langenbeck** (◘ Fig. 4.49).

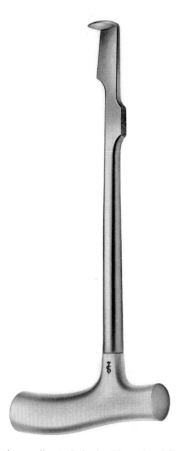

◘ Fig. 4.46 Chisel according to Lebsche. (Aesculap AG, with kind permission)

If bones are to be cut, saws or bone shears are used. The cutting instruments are also called bone forceps, they can also be used to remove splintered bone parts (◘ Fig. 4.50). In the jaws, two ground cutting edges meet and cut through strong cortical structures. The working part can be straight, curved or bent at right angles, depending on the bone shape and location.

Luer's gouge forceps are the best known bone forceps for removing bone fragments and cartilage (◘ Fig. 4.51). The jaws of these forceps are shaped like a curette, but the edges of the curette are sharply ground so that cartilage tissue can be removed. This instrument exists in many variations and modifications. Comparable forceps are named after **Olivecrona**, **Jansen** or **Frykholm.**

4

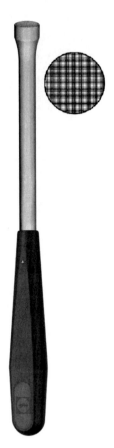

🔲 **Fig. 4.47**   Tamper. (Aesculap AG, with kind permission)

Meniscus and Cartilage Forceps

The meniscus forceps are used to resect capsular remnants or to grasp cartilage. In their jaws are strong, sharp teeth which hold the cartilage firmly so that it can then be resected with a scalpel (🔲 Fig. 4.52).

Reposition Forceps

In order to secure the repositioning result after a fracture until the implants have been inserted for stabilization, there are a variety of reposition forceps. They encompass the bone shape, therefore the forceps for long bones have a round jaw shape, for flat or smaller bones as well as for cartilage structures two pointed jaw ends, shaped e.g. like a pointed towel clamp (🔲 Fig. 4.53). All reposition forceps are available with and without ratchet or with locking screws that allow slow release of fixation (🔲 Fig. 4.54).

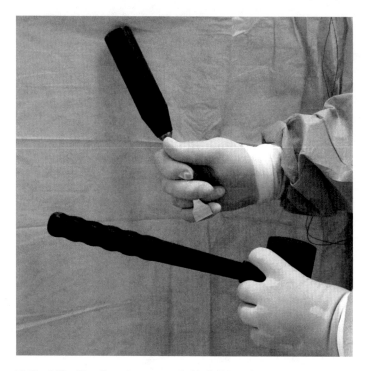

□ Fig. 4.48   Handing a hammer and chisel. (Photo by Margret Liehn)

There are many reposition forceps, which cannot all be named and shown here. They are identical in their application; the shape of the jaws indicates the bones to which they can be applied (□ Fig. 4.55).

4.3.7 Wire Instruments

To secure a cerclage, appropriate wire pliers are required, some of which are known from the craftmanship. Flat nose pliers are used to grasp and pull a wire, side cutters are used to cut a wire, and needle nose pliers, also known as round nose pliers, are used to twist the ends of the wire and to sink the ends of the wire. All these pliers are not lockable, because they have to be opened and moved frequently during use.

A flat-nose pliers has two flattened, grained jaw ends that can grip the wire firmly (□ Fig. 4.56).

Depending on the diameter of the wire ends to be cut, the side cutter is shaped. The two strong, sharp working ends of the side cutter allow the wire to be cut (□ Fig. 4.57).

Both working ends of the needle-nose pliers are rounded and taper to a point (□ Fig. 4.58). This allows wire ends to be twisted against each other and bent over so that they can be

4

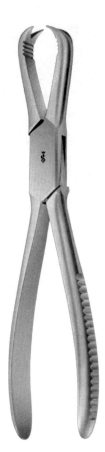

◘ **Fig. 4.49**   Bone holding forceps according to Langenbeck. (Aesculap AG, with kind permission)

countersunk, thus avoiding any risk of injury to surrounding structures. Thinner wires can be cut with wire cutters, one blade of which is serrated to prevent the wire from slipping off (◘ Fig. 4.59).

To tension wires, pliers can also be used (◘ Fig. 4.60), so called "**wire-twister**". In their jaws they have a strong grained profile which prevents the wire from slipping off.

If the cerclage wire is difficult to tighten with the above-mentioned pliers, a wire tensioner can be used, which by its mechanism causes tension on the wire by squeezing the branches together (◘ Fig. 4.61).

▪ **Handling**

All forceps are handed closed (◘ Fig. 4.62). The nurse has to grasp the end of the working part and place it in the surgeon's hand in such a way that the surgeon not has to turn the forceps

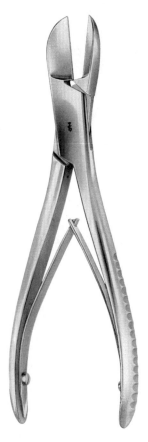

■ **Fig. 4.50** Bone cutting forceps according to Lister. (Aesculap AG, with kind permission)

and can use them immediately in the correct position. To do this, the scrub nurse must know where and for which purpose the forceps are needed. The mouth of the instrument points to the bone, the handle to the surgeon's hand.

If parts of bone or cartilage are resected, it must be known or, if necessary, asked whether the removed material should be given for histological examination, can be discarded or should be reused.

4.3.8 Drilling Systems

In order to be able to use screws in and on the bone, drilling systems are required with which the hard cortical bone can be drilled. The machines have different drives, depending on the manufacturer. They can be driven by compressed air or electri-

4

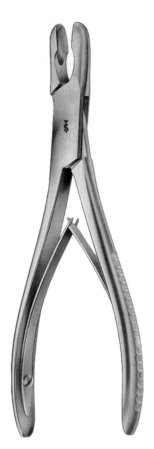

◘ Fig. 4.51   Gouge forceps according to Luer. (Aesculap AG, with kind permission)

cally. If the machine is used with a compressed air hose or electric cable, it must be ensured that the hose is long enough to guarantee sterility.

However, the standard of most manufacturers is to insert a charged battery into the machine. These batteries cannot be sterilized, so a large template is placed on the opened drill (◘ Fig. 4.63), the circulating nurse inserts the suitable battery and removes the template. The scrub nurse closes the machine and it is ready to work. The inserted battery changes the weight of the machine as well as its center of gravity. This must be taken into account during working.

The appropriate twist drills and/or thread cutters for osteosynthesis can be inserted into the machines. The drills have a snap lock for this purpose, which is opened with the left hand so that the desired twist drill can be inserted. The tight fit of the inserted drill must be tested before it is presented to the

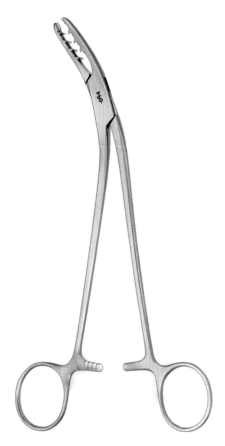

Fig. 4.52 Cartilage forceps according to Bircher-Ganske. (Aesculap AG, with kind permission)

surgeon. Some manufacturers have a rotary mechanism for inserting the drill attachments.

Another possibility for inserting drill attachments is the **Jacob's chuck** (◘ Fig. 4.64). This chuck is opened manually so far that the drill can be inserted. The drill attachment is fixed with a **Jacob's key** (◘ Fig. 4.65).

Since bones are so hard that a scalpel cannot be used to cut through bone, a saw is often used in addition to the bone cutting pliers mentioned above. They are normally used with an air-powered drill. The saw blades are adapted to the bone to be sawn through and inserted into the corresponding chuck with a suitable key.

Those saws are named as the "oscillating saw", which means that the saw blade moves in an oscillating motion by the motor, thus cutting through the cortical bone.

4

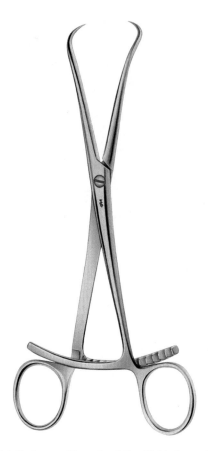

🔲 **Fig. 4.53**   Patella forceps. (Aesculap AG, with kind permission)

■ Handling

After the drill has been prepared, the required drill attachments are made ready. The scrub nurse knows the planned osteosynthesis and the needed implant system. The diameter of the twist drill depends on the core diameter of the desired screw and varies with different systems; the same applies to the thread cutters. Here we can only refer to the corresponding surgical textbooks and manufacturer's manuals.

Perforators (🔲 Fig. 4.66) or diamond burrs (🔲 Fig. 4.67) may also be required for smoothing or reaming bone.

The surgeon gets the prepared machine in such a way that he can activate the trigger immediately. For this purpose, the nurse must grip the machine in such a way that the drill attachment cannot bend (🔲 Fig. 4.68). In addition, accidental triggering of the drill mechanism could injure the nurse. The weight of the machine causes it to be gripped above the drill trigger.

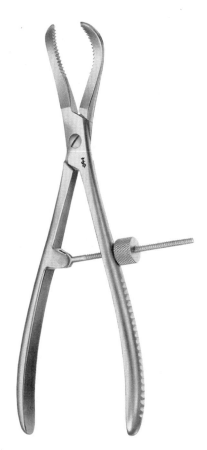

□ Fig. 4.54 Reposition forceps with locking screw. (Aesculap AG, with kind permission)

When the machine is not in use, it must **never** be placed on the patient to prevent injuries from accidental triggering. Either the drill is placed on the instrument table or a drill pocket is fixed to this table in which the machine can be placed. If there is a possibility on the system to turn off the drill, this should always be done; before handing it to the surgeon, make sure that the mechanism is released again.

Any drilling or milling on a bone will cause the bone material to become hot. Heat on the bone can lead to necrosis, so it is essential to cool the bones while drilling or milling. After the surgeon grasps the drill, the assistant is handed a syringe filled with irrigation fluid with a tip cannula.

Some manufacturers have the option on their drills to run a flush via an infusion system. In practice, this is usually cum-

4

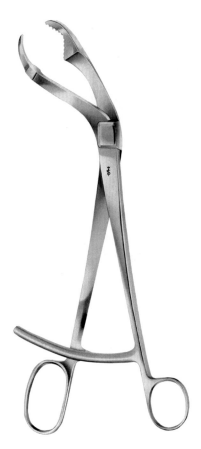

◻ **Fig. 4.55**   Reposition forceps according to Verbrugge. (Aesculap AG, with kind permission)

bersome, time-consuming and is therefore often not set up. The different systems can be operated by manual triggering or by foot switch.

The instrument handling in traumatology and orthopedics is very diverse and always manufacturer-specific. There is usually a matching implantation instrument set for the different implants. Implants only fit if the correctly prepared instrument set is used.

> ❯ Basic rules are that instruments and implants must fit together, systems from different manufacturers cannot be mixed. The plates and screws used must be made of the same material. Screws and plates that have already been used must not be used a second time.

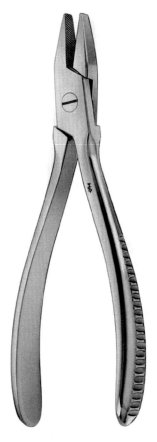

☐ Fig. 4.56 Flat-nose pliers. (Aesculap AG, with kind permission)

4.4 **Gynaecological Instruments**

In the gynaecology department, basic instruments such as scissors, forceps and needle holders are also used, the function has already been described. As in the other specialties, there are special instruments that are used according to their function. Again, there will be different names for the special instruments needed. For example, the industry offers a wide variety of grasping forceps with different special names for grasping the uterus, so only a small excerpt can be mentioned here as well.

In the case of working in the gynaecological OR theatre, it should be borne in mind that the procedures are either performed abdominally, in which case all the rules already men-

4

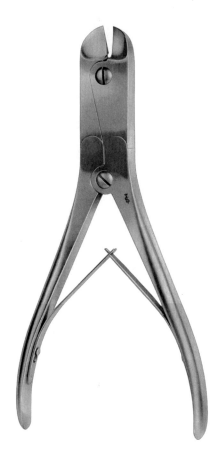

◘ Fig. 4.57 Side cutter, front and lateral cutting action. (Aesculap AG, with kind permission)

tioned for instruments apply. However, if the procedure is performed via a vaginal approach, the angle of presenting the instruments changes, as the scrub nurse often stands diagonally behind the seated surgeon or is also seated.

To ensure the sterility of the instrument, the instrument passed the right side of the surgeon's upper arm. Then it is necessary to consider how the instrument is used, which anatomical structure the bend should follow. Accordingly, the instrument is in the hand of the nurse.

Minimally invasive surgery is also used for many gynaecological procedures. The handling and presenting is the same as discussed in ▶ Sect. 4.2.

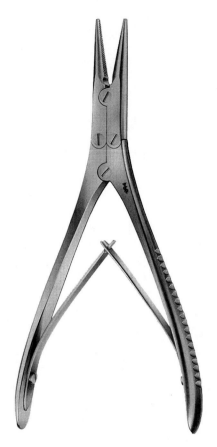

■ **Fig. 4.58** Needle-nose pliers. (Fa. Aesculap AG, with friendly permission)

4.4.1 **Vaginal Specula**

The word speculum (plural: specula) comes from Latin and means something like mirror. This term covers all instruments that are channel- or tube-shaped. They are inserted into natural orifices (rectal speculum, nasal speculum).

In gynaecology, differently shaped specula are used to open and inspect the vaginal vault. This allows the surgeon to inspect the vagina, identify the cervix and visualize the portio.

Vaginal specula are available in hand-held and self-retaining versions. The specula are adapted to the anatomical proportions of the patient, so that they are available in many sizes. They are used for all vaginal procedures. Some specula

4

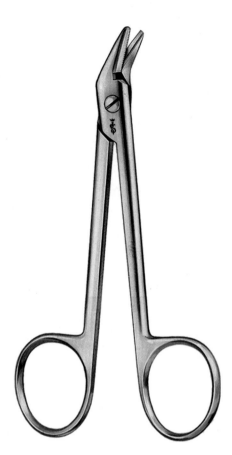

◘ Fig. 4.59 Wire cutting scissors. (Aesculap AG, with kind permission)

can have a detachable weight so that they act as a self-holder. The **Kristeller** vaginal speculum is a vaginal inserter without a self-holding device (◘ Fig. 4.69).

A distinction is made between an anterior, posterior and a lateral blade, depending on whether the anterior or posterior vaginal vault is to be represented. The posterior blade is a gutter speculum because of its shape, it has a gutter for draining off fluids and collecting secretions. Since it is inserted "below", it is also called lower blade in the manufacturers' catalogues, the flat shaped blade is called anterior or upper blade.

The **Scherback** vaginal speculum is available with different blades and groove. By attaching a weight to the lower blade, it functions as a self-retaining speculum (◘ Fig. 4.70).

The vaginal speculum according to **Breisky** is curved differently and allows vaginal adjustment in all directions and is

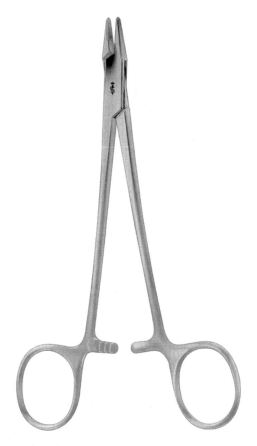

■ **Fig. 4.60**   Wire twister. (Fa. Aesculap AG, with kind permission)

therefore often used laterally. The blades are available in long and short, the designations for these vary in the operating theatres, they are frequently designated as a lateral blade numbered 1–5 (■ Fig. 4.71).

The **Doyen** speculum is quite wide and is often used as a lower blade during vaginal surgery to provide a clear view of the situs (■ Fig. 4.72).

All vaginal specula are available in smaller versions for use in pediatric surgery.

■ Handling

Vaginal specula are always applied moist in order to prevent the vaginal mucosa from drying out even if the instruments are left in place for a longer period of time. The scrub nurse

4

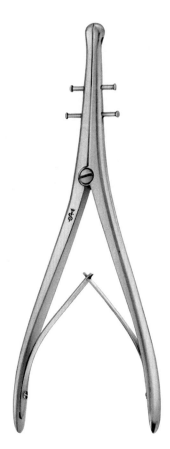

◘ Fig. 4.61 Wire tightening and twisting forceps according to Demel. (Aesculap AG, with kind permission)

knows the names and the field of application of the individual specula and, if necessary, the in-house size designation.

A speculum has a slightly curved handle and the respective blade (with or without groove). The nurse always grasps the instrument by the blade, holding it horizontally so that the surgeon can grasp the vertically upward or downward handle and insert the speculum immediately (◘ Fig. 4.73).

4.4.2 Uterine Dilators

A dilator is an instrument used to dilate a canal, the name "bougie" is also common. These instruments are made of

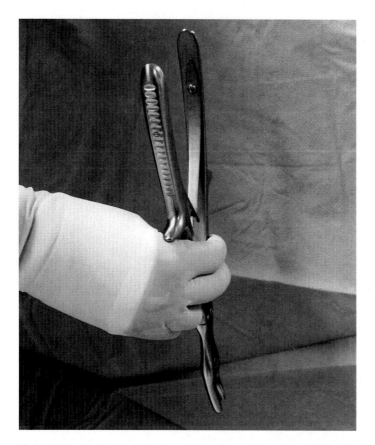

Fig. 4.62 Application of a bone forceps according to Luer. (Photo by Margret Liehn)

metal or plastic and have a rounded or conical point. They are available for gradual dilation in ascending diameter, which is measured in "Charrière".

Before uterine curettes can be inserted into the uterus for scraping, the cervix must be dilated. Metal are used for this purpose. These uterine dilators are available straight or slightly S-shaped (**Figs. 4.74 and 4.75**).

■ Handling

Dilators should also be moistened so that they can glide in the mucous membrane of the cervix (NaCl 0.9% corrodes the surface alloy of an instrument and promotes rust formation).

A dilator is grasped by the nurse at the blunt end and held horizontally so that the surgeon can insert it immediately. The

4

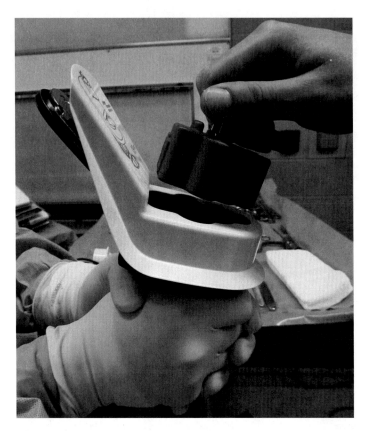

◨ **Fig. 4.63** Drilling machine with template for inserting the battery. The battery is still in the hand of the circulating nurse. (Photo by Margret Liehn)

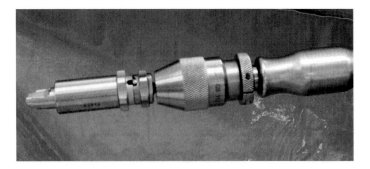

◨ **Fig. 4.64** Jacob's chuck with trepan clamped in a drilling machine. (Photo by Margret Liehn)

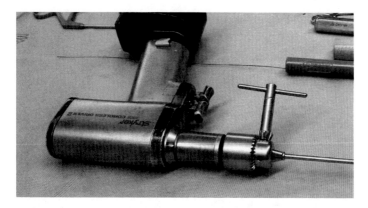

Fig. 4.65 Jacob's key in use. (Photo by Margret Liehn)

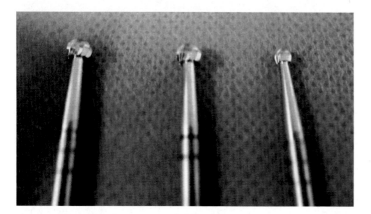

Fig. 4.66 Perforator. (Photo by Margret Liehn)

bougie is then passed on in ascending diameter until the cervix has been dilated sufficiently for the insertion of a curette, for example.

4.4.3 Uterine Curettes

The word originally comes from French, so "curettage" is also a correct term meaning scraping. Uterine curettes are used in gynaecology for scraping the lining of the uterus (endometrium). It is important to know whether this scraping is carried out on a non-pregnant or a pregnant uterus, because this determines whether sharp or blunt curettes are used.

4

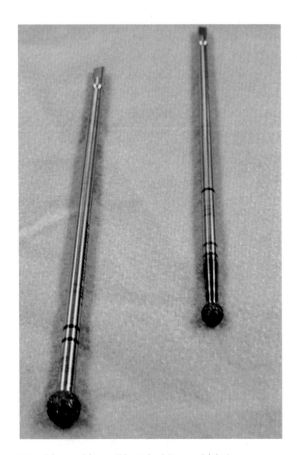

Fig. 4.67 Diamond burr. (Photo by Margret Liehn)

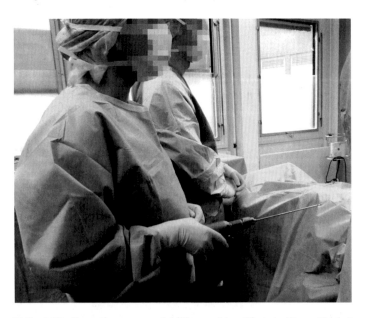

Fig. 4.68 Presenting a prepared drilling machine. (Photo by Margret Liehn)

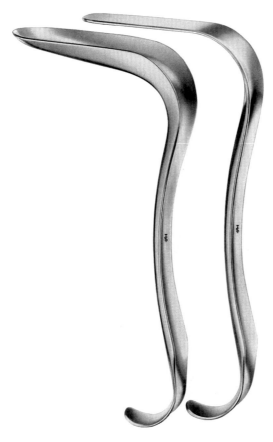

■ **Fig. 4.69** Vaginal speculum according to Kristeller. (Aesculap AG, with kind permission)

The instruments are available straight or slightly bent in the working end, fixed or slightly flexible. The **blunt curette** is a long, straight instrument with a handle and an open spoon-like working end which is not ground. Depending on the size of the uterus, curettes are used to scrape the uterus, e.g., in postabortion conditions (■ Fig. 4.76) or to terminate an existing pregnancy. Since the uterus is very soft due to pregnancy and there is a risk of perforation, only blunt ovum curettes are used (■ Fig. 4.77).

The sharp curette is shaped in the same way as the blunt one; it is available straight or slightly bent, firm or slightly flexible. Again, the different sizes of instrument are used according to the extent of the uterus (■ Figs. 4.78 and 4.79). The instrument is used for abrasion in cases of suspected cervical or corpus carcinoma.

Note: In a **fractionated abrasion,** the cervix is first scraped and only then dilated. This prevents any tumour cells that may be present from entering the corpus.

4

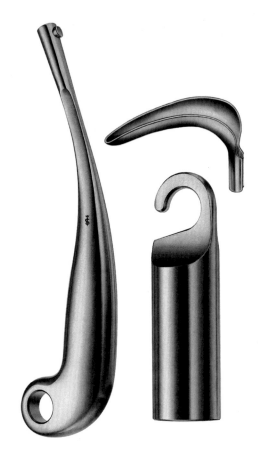

◻ **Fig. 4.70**   Vaginal speculum according to Scherback (with detachable weight). (Aesculap AG, with kind permission)

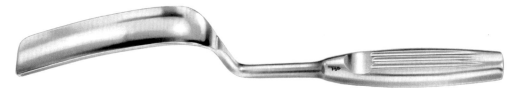

◻ **Fig. 4.71**   Vaginal speculum according to Breisky. (Aesculap AG, with kind permission)

■ **Handling**

The scrub nurse must always check whether the uterine curette is sharp or blunt before passing it to the surgeon. You can run your thumb over the opening; the difference between a sharp curette and a blunt one can be clearly felt. The nurse grips the instrument at the working end and places the handle horizontally in the surgeon's hand.

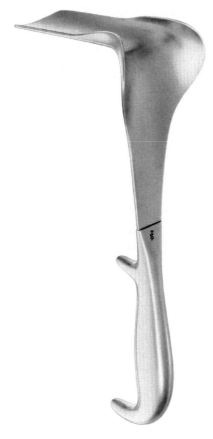

◘ Fig. 4.72 Vaginal speculum according to Doyen. (Aesculap AG, with kind permission)

Uterine Probe

A long, curved, graduated probe is attached to a grooved handle and ends in a small ball (◘ Fig. 4.80). This measuring probe can be used to determine the length of the uterus. This determines how far the uterine curettes may be inserted.

Note: Do not use a probe in a pregnant uterus, as the risk of perforation is serious! A probe with a thick ball at the end may be used.

■ Handling

All instruments that are used vaginally should be moistened before use to facilitate insertion vaginally or through the cervix. The uterine probe is grasped by the ball and held horizontally so that it can be inserted immediately.

4

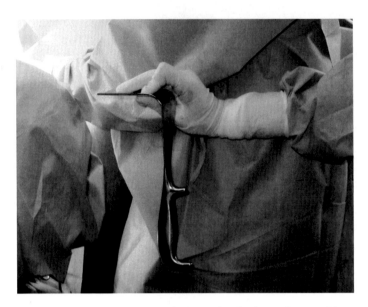

◘ Fig. 4.73 Presentation of a vaginal speculum by the scrub nurse. (Photo by Margret Liehn)

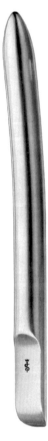

◘ Fig. 4.74 Straight Hegar dilator. (Aesculap AG, with kind permission)

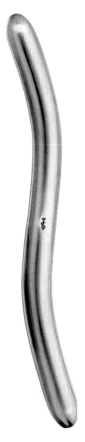

Fig. 4.75 Curved Hegar dilator. (Aesculap AG, with kind permission)

4.4.4 Clamps and Forceps

Many clamps and forceps used in gynaecology are similar to those described in the chapter on abdominal surgery (▶ Sect. 4.1), especially organ grasping forceps. Only a few that have been developed specifically for gynaecology are mentioned here.

Ovum Forceps

These forceps consist of two parts which are screwed together (◘ Fig. 4.81). They are often slightly curved and have an oval opening at the front to ensure a constant view of the blood supply to the ovaries. For grasping, the forceps have two rings into which the thumb and middle finger can be placed to open the forceps. The cross-grooving on the inside of the oval openings allows the ovaries to be grasped without causing damage. The forceps are used to grasp, hold or lift the ovaries to allow access to the surgical area. These ovum forceps are available with and without a lock.

Alternatively, there is the **Kelly** clamp without a ratchet.

4

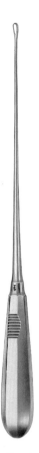

■ **Fig. 4.76** Ovum curette according to Recamier. (Aesculap AG, with kind permission)

Parametrium Clamps

The parametrium clamps are used in abdominal hysterectomy (■ Fig. 4.82). They are powerful grasping forceps, slightly curved. They have a longitudinal groove in the working parts which fixes the tissue but does not injure it.

Alternatively, the hysterectomy clamp according to **Wertheim** is available, which looks similar. This clamp is also available in straight, curved and angled form. Strong clamps with two teeth (surgically traumatic forceps) at the ends of the jaws for tight closure of the forceps are also popular hysterectomy clamps. The jaw profile is not serrated longitudinally or transversely, but diagonally to prevent tissue slippage. This allows the adnexal ducts and the ovarian artery to be grasped. These grasping forceps are designed to be strong enough to prevent the vessels from slipping off.

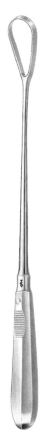

◻ Fig. 4.77 Blunt curette according to Bumm. (Aesculap AG, with kind permission)

Tenaculum Forceps

The different tenaculum forceps are used for abdominal procedures to grasp the uterus or fibroids (◻ Figs. 4.83 and 4.84). In vaginal procedures, the tenaculum forceps with teethed tips are used to grasp the cervix (portio). In the jaws of the forceps are one, two, four, or six teeth on each side, provided for grasping and holding, depending on the size of the uterus.

Alternatively, tenaculum forceps according to **Czerny**, **Museux**, **Martin** or **Braun** are available.

■ Handling

The OR scrub nurse grasps the forceps with the right hand at the working end, the bending of the instrument follows the hand over the closed fingers. The surgeon places the instrument in the palm of the hand. He then grips the rings with his thumb and middle finger.

4

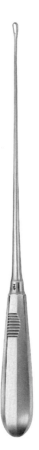

◨ **Fig. 4.78** Sharp uterine curette according to Recamier. (Aesculap AG, with kind permission)

In the case of vaginal access, the instrument is placed in the slightly raised hand of the surgeon from above at an oblique angle. The bending of the instrument already follows the anatomical structure of the layer to be grasped during the approach (◨ Fig. 4.85).

4.4.5 **Scissors**

In gynaecology, scissors are often preferred that are strong at the end of the jaws and curved additionally at the handle in the lower third to better reach the angle in the woman's small pelvis for depositing the vaginal part from the uterus (◨ Fig. 4.86).

■ **Handling**

Here, too, the presenting of the instruments depends on the position of the nurse. In the case of an abdominal approach, the nurse is usually facing the surgeon. The instrument is to be

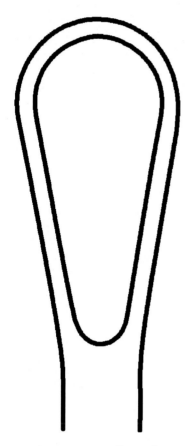

□ Fig. 4.79 Sharp uterine curette according to Sims. (Aesculap AG, with kind permission)

grasped at the working end in such a way that the bend at the mouth of the scissors curves over the index finger of the instrument user.

In the case of a vaginal approach, the scrub nurse must rotate the hand with the instrument so that the surgeon can grasp the scissors in such a way that the curve of the scissors' jaws follows the structure to be cut.

4.4.6 Special Gynaecological Instruments

In every gynaecological department there are special instruments, of which only one can be mentioned here because of the variety.

Hysteroscope

The word "hystera" comes from the Greek and means uterus, "scopie" means mirroring. Hysteroscopy (uterus endoscopy)

4

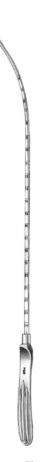

☐ **Fig. 4.80**   Uterus probe according to Sims. (Aesculap AG, with kind permission)

means viewing the uterine cavity using optical instruments. The image of the cavity is transferred to a monitor. The indication for a hysteroscopy can be diagnostic as well as therapeutic.

Before curettage, hysteroscopy is often performed to avoid scraping in an unknown space. After disinfection and adjustment of the vagina by means of specula, the hysteroscope, an illumination rod with a diameter of approximately 3.5 mm, is inserted. In order to unfold the uterine cavity, warmed "Purisole solution" is introduced.

NaCl must not be used during a hysteroscopy because of the use of an HF device, as this can cause burns.

The instrument is connected to a video system and transmits the image of the uterine cavity in multiple magnification on the screen, so that a decision can be made quickly about the progress of the procedure. Polypus can be removed via the hysteroscope, tissue samples can be taken for cancer diagnosis or a visual diagnosis of the mucous membrane can be made.

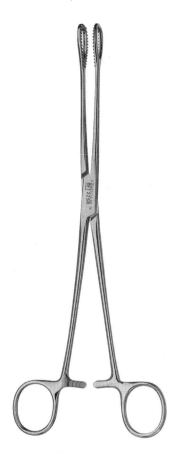

☐ **Fig. 4.81** Tissue grasping forceps according to Förster-Ballenger. (Aesculap AG, with kind permission)

The hysteroscope consists of two parts, an optic and a shaft (☐ Fig. 4.87). The instrument must be assembled prior to surgery. All connections, light guide cables and irrigation tubing are checked and connected only after the hysteroscope has been placed in the uterus.

Many gynaecological operations can be performed laparoscopically. In many cases, the instruments are similar to those presented in ▶ Sect. 4.2.

4.5 Urological Instruments

In urology, the familiar basic and abdominal instruments are required and, in the case of incisional operations, some special instruments which are presented here. However, many procedures are performed transurethrally and here other instruments are used than those discussed so far.

4

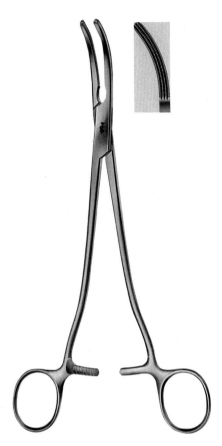

■ **Fig. 4.82**   Hysterectomy clamp according to Heany. (Aesculap AG, with kind permission)

4.5.1 **TURP and TURB Instruments**

The abbreviation TURP stands for transurethral resection of the prostate, which means that tissue is removed from the bladder or prostate through the urethra. For this purpose, an instrument with a lumen is inserted into the bladder through the urethra and connected to a light source and a monitor so that the surgeon can see the surgical field on the monitor. The diseased tissue is then removed by high-frequency current, with a loop electrode.

In advance, a urethrotome is inserted into the urethra to incise it at its narrow point. This can be done under visual control as a urethrotomy according to Sachse or "blindly" as a urethrotomy according to Otis (■ Fig. 4.88). The urethral knife is integrated into the instrument and is manually extended by the surgeon when the constriction is reached.

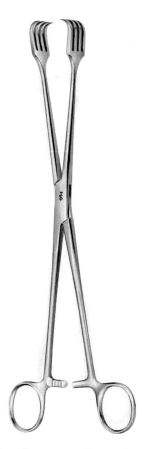

◘ Fig. 4.83 Tenaculum forceps according to Aesculap-Pratt. (Aesculap AG, with kind permission)

If tissue is to be removed from the prostate or bladder the instrument is called resectoscope (◘ Fig. 4.89). An optic is inserted into this resectoscope to enable vision, irrigation fluid is supplied and drained via various working channels and the individual resection instruments are introduced.

If work is carried out in a space filled with liquid by means of high-frequency current, this liquid must not conduct electricity under any circumstances, therefore saline solution or water is not possible. The solution must be electrolyte-free, which is why "Purisole" (Fresenius-Kabi) is often used.

■ **Handling**

As the patient is positioned in lithotomy position for these procedures, the surgeon sits between the raised legs. The same rules of instrumentation apply here as were addressed for the vaginal procedures. The scrub nurse stands at the back of the surgeon and passes the instruments past the surgeon's right arm.

4

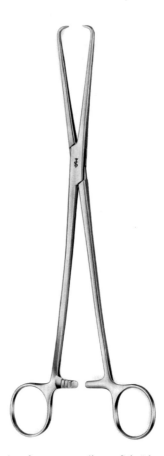

◻ **Fig. 4.84**   Tenaculum forceps according to Schröder. (Aesculap AG, with kind permission)

In advance, the individual instruments must be assembled. This must be practiced beforehand, because each manufacturer prefers its own mechanics. The instruments are assembled and it must be checked whether the individual mechanics function smoothly, only then an instrument can be used. All required additional instruments are ready in standardized form.

The nurse must grasp the instrument by its working part and hand it at an angle with the handle pointing upwards so that it can be inserted immediately into the urethra. All transurethrally required instruments are handed in this form.

Many urological procedures are performed laparoscopically, using instruments similar to those described in ▶ Sect. 4.2, with a few additional instruments for stone retrieval. These look like small baskets or spoons and can pick up stones

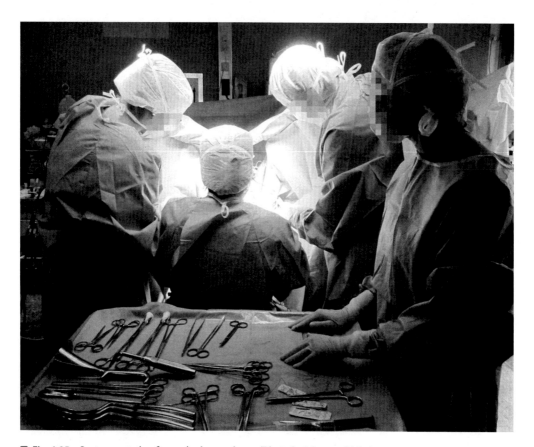

◘ Fig. 4.85 Instrumentation for vaginal procedures. (Photo by Margret Liehn)

and retrieve them externally through a trocar. The instrumentation does not change.

Conventional Procedures in Urology

If the operation is performed through an incision, basic and laparotomy instruments are used.

4.5.2 Prostate and Bladder

Due to the special anatomical conditions, e.g. in the small pelvis, the retractors must be long and narrow and have a relatively acute angle (◘ Fig. 4.90).

Space for surgical procedures is very limited in the small pelvis, so self-retaining systems are preferred (◘ Fig. 4.91).

Retractors, grasping forceps and dissecting clamps are often angled in the handle to keep access to the prostate clear (◘ Fig. 4.92).

4

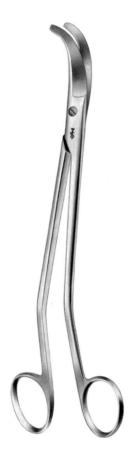

◘ Fig. 4.86 Uterine scissors according to Bozemann. (Aesculap AG, with kind permission)

4.5.3 **Kidneys**

If surgery is performed on the kidney, it is usually due to a tumor or stone disease. If a kidney is removed, the required clamps must grip tightly to avoid severe bleeding, the blood supply must only be interrupted temporarily, and the delicate vascular structures at the renal hilus must not be destroyed by the clamping. The same applies to clamps that are intended to grip the ureter.

This means that the clamps have atraumatic striations and a bend in the working part which ensures a clear view. Special clamps for urology are used here (◘ Fig. 4.93) or atraumatic clamps known from intestinal or vascular surgery, such as the **Satinsky clamp** (▶ Chap. 3, ◘ Fig. 3.40).

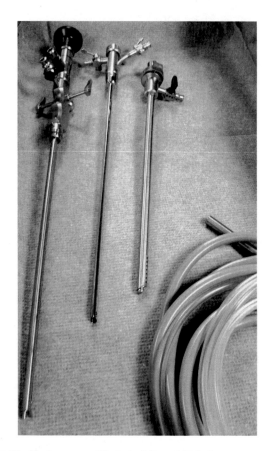

Fig. 4.87 Hysteroscope. (Photo by Margret Liehn)

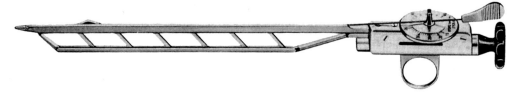

Fig. 4.88 Urethrotome according to Otis. (Karl Storz Company, with kind permission)

Comparable would be the kidney clamp according to **Stille**, which is not shown here. In order to work on the kidney hilus, a bending of the jaws as with the **Satinsky clamp** or an angulation as with the **Wertheim clamp** is required to maintain visibility.

4

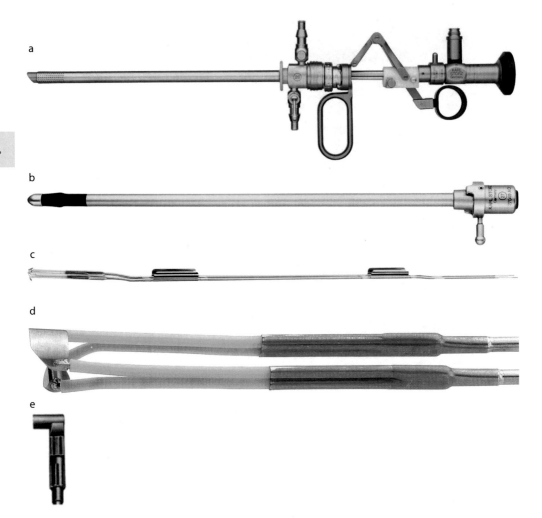

■ **Fig. 4.89 a–e** Electroresection instrument. **a** Resectoscope with inserted optics and Teflon-covered shaft with central stopcock. **b** Atraumatic spreader obturator according to Leusch for the shaft covering the sharp-edged shaft end. **c** Loop electrode. **d** Electrode variants: hook probe at the top, coagulation electrode with ball roller at the bottom. **e** Connection of the electrode to the high-frequency guide cable on the electrotome. (Karl Storz, with kind permission)

Kidney stone forceps are needed to grasp, hold and remove a stone (◘ Fig. 4.94). To accommodate all anatomical regions, they are available with a wide variety of bends in the working part. They are not lockable so that the surgeon can feel how firmly the stone must be held in the forceps; a ratchet could destroy the stone by too firm pressure and thus leave stone concretions in the situs.

■ **Handling**

Handling of the instruments in conventional urology differs in presenting instruments for transurethral surgery (▶ Sect. 4.5.1). Here, the scrub nurse faces the surgeon. The surgeon stands on the side of the patient on which the findings were diagnosed.

All instruments are grasped at the working part, the bend follows the anatomical structure where the instrument is to be inserted.

In pelvic surgery, it is often difficult for the surgeon to have an unobstructed view of the situs. Therefore, it may happen in the beginning that the corresponding instrument is not handed in the needed shape. The scrub nurse has to follow closely what the surgeon does with the instrument, because if he has to turn the instrument in his hand before it can be inserted, this should be taken into account the next time it is presented.

4.6 Vascular Surgery Instruments

Vascular surgery procedures are performed in special departments, nevertheless some of the required instruments are available in every department and must be known. In order to perform interventions on the vascular system, some basic rules must be observed.

The structure of veins and arteries must be known, as this provides insight into the clamps and suture material required. When a vessel is to be clamped, whether for placement of a

4

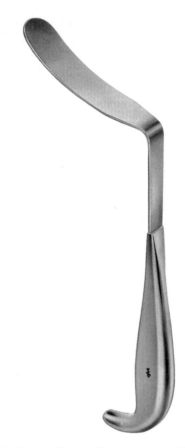

◻ **Fig. 4.90**   Bladder spatula according to Legueu. (Aesculap AG, with kind permission)

bypass, an interposition device, a vein graft, or a vascular prosthesis, the scrub nurse must know the correct clamp, be able to determine the suture material with the correct needle shape and select the appropriate needle holder.

The requirement for instruments used to grasp, clamp and unclamp vessels is always that of atraumatic striation and soft elastic locking. Veins have no musculature, so they are even more sensitive to traumatic forceps and hard grasping clamps than arteries. Therefore, atraumatic forceps (▶ Sect. 3.1.2) are used during surgical interventions on the vascular system.

The size of the clamp depends on the caliber of the vessel. On the aorta, the clamp must hold a greater resistance than on the femoral artery. The shape of the entire instrument depends on the access to the vessel, especially the bends in the branches correspond to the surgical site.

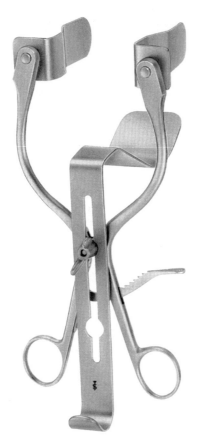

◻ Fig. 4.91 Bladder spreader according to Millin. (Aesculap AG, with kind permission)

4.6.1 **Vascular Clamps**

Many vascular clamps have already been named and described in ▶ Sect. 3.1.4 because they can also be used as bowel clamps.

In addition, there are arterial or vascular clamps that have been specially developed for vascular surgery. These clamps always have atraumatically profiled jaws; they are grained, grooved, smooth, cross serrated or teethed. Many clamps are named after this atraumatic graining, depending on which vascular surgeon preferred the profile: **De Bakey** (longitudinally grooved with the finest teeth, cross serrated) or **Cooley** (similar, the grooving is more plastically arranged).

4

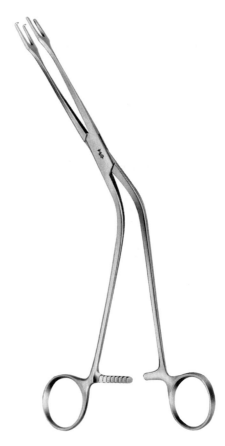

◻ **Fig. 4.92** Prostate grasping forceps according to Millin. (Aesculap AG, with kind permission)

In some departments there are other **forceps** or clamps, also with an atraumatic longitudinally grooved or grained jaw profile, the name being that of the manufacturing company. **Cooley**'s clamps are considered vascular clamps (◻ Fig. 4.95). They are available with variously angled (30°, 60°, 90°, etc.) jaws and an atraumatic serration that permits grasping of tissue without crushing.

The vascular clamps according to **De Bakey** have a special atraumatic serration developed by him, they can be used as vascular clamps but also as ligature clamps or intestinal clamps (◻ Fig. 4.96). The branches are bent and the jaws are curved in different ways.

In surgery, often only the angle of the clamp is used, 45° or 90° angled clamps, curved or S-shaped clamps.

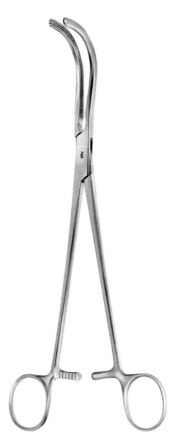

☐ Fig. 4.93 Kidney clamp according to Guyon. (Aesculap AG, with kind permission)

Vascular clamps either lock resiliently or have an elastic-clamping ratchet to avoid trauma in the vessel lumen. This defined closing pressure is expressed in grams and often marked with artery or vein. If the clamps are applied manually, they have a grooved handle so that the surgeon can grip precisely and never slip off the clamp (☐ Figs. 4.97 and 4.98).

For very fine vessels, micro-bulldog clamps are used which, because of their size, can no longer be applied directly by hand but are placed using clip application forceps (☐ Figs. 4.99 and 4.100).

Comparable vascular clamps are named after **De Bakey**, **Glover** or **Dieffenbach**.

4

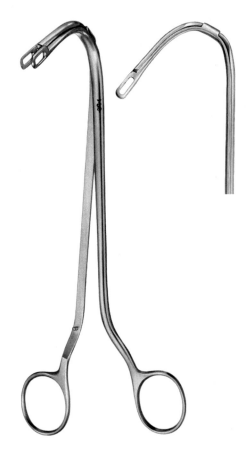

■ **Fig. 4.94** Kidney stone forceps according to Randall. (Aesculap AG, with kind permission)

Handling of Vascular Clamps

❯ Every scrub nurse must know the procedure and it must be absolutely clear what could happen if the wrong instrument is used.

Based on the surgical site, the nurse can choose the length and shape of the required clamp. The clamp is grasped at the mouth, the bend of the mouth usually follows the curvature of the scrub nurses right hand, to be held diagonally and handed over to the surgeon (■ Figs. 4.101 and 4.102).

  When presenting a mini - bulldog in the applicator, it must be borne in mind that the clamp is not fixed in the forceps and must therefore not fall out of the applicator on the way to the situs. Of course, all clamps are counted pre-, intra- and post-operatively.

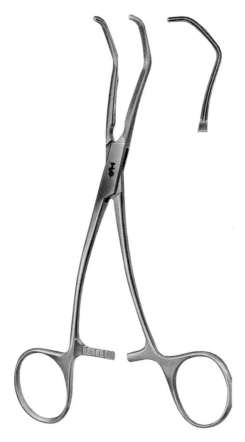

🔲 Fig. 4.95 Vascular clamp according to Cooley. (Aesculap AG, with kind permission)

4.6.2 **Vascular Spatulas (Dissectors)**

Calcium deposits, for example, can become lodged in the lumen of a vessel. In order to remove these bluntly and gently, a dissector is often used (🔲 Figs. 4.103 and 4.104). Dissect means to split, to separate. A dissection can be performed with an instrument, but also by means of a water jet, ultrasound and other media. Vascular dissectors are blunt or sharp, consist of a handle and the working end. As a rule, the blunt dissectors are used in vascular surgery (in ENT, the sharp dissectors are used to peel the tonsils from their bed).

The working end is slightly bent up, the handle stronger with a grooved surface. Dissectors with a double ended working part are also used. Check, if both ends are blunt or that one is blunt and the other sharp (▶ Sect. 4.3.1).

4

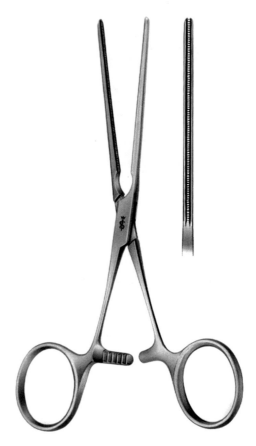

☐ **Fig. 4.96** Vascular clamp according to De Bakey. (Aesculap AG, with kind permission)

Handling

The instrument is grasped at its working end, with the bent-up surface pointing into the vessel. The dissector is held at an angle and handed over to the surgeon with the working surface first.

4.6.3 **Shears**

In vascular surgery, very differently bent and angled scissors (☐ Figs. 4.105 and 4.106) are used in order to be able to cut precisely in and on the vessel. The **Potts de Martell** angled scissors are used to open a vessel longitudinally after a stab incision; the angle can vary. Straight, pointed scissors are preferred for transecting a vessel. For difficult access situs, the branches may be curved in an S-shape or C-shape.

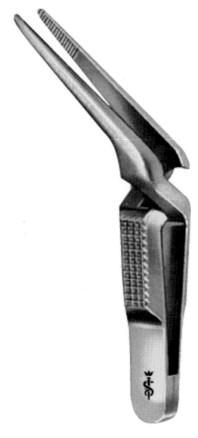

◘ Fig. 4.97 Bulldog clamp according to De Bakey-Hess. (Aesculap AG, with kind permission)

■ **Handling**

The presenting rules are given in ▶ Sect. 4.6.1. The scrub nurse is aware of the intended use and is able to present the needed scissors according to the situs.

4.6.4 **Nerve and Vessel Hooks**

To take a vessel or a nerve, there is a blunt hook, either bent 90° or with a probe ending. This hook can be led under the vessel and detach it from the surrounding structures if necessary. Some have a small probe end, others are just rounded (◘ Figs. 4.107 and 4.108).

4

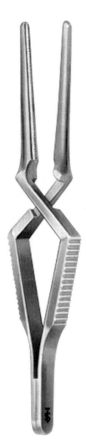

◘ **Fig. 4.98**   Bulldog clamp according to De Bakey. (Aesculap AG, with kind permission)

4.6.5 Set for Tunneling and Pulling through E.G. Vascular Grafts

The last instrument to be mentioned here is one that tunnels tissue, e.g. to guide a prepared vein or a vascular graft through soft tissue (◘ Fig. 4.109). This is done by spreading the soft tissue, inserting the tunneling tube in the opposite direction, and pulling the vein through. In many departments, a slightly curved dressing forceps is used instead.

Many other instruments are used in vascular surgery which are not mentioned here. It is essential to get to know the instruments and to practice their determined use, their handling and their names via surgical lessons and textbooks and above all in one's own surgical department. Every trained colleague and every surgeon will certainly be happy to fill in gaps in knowledge.

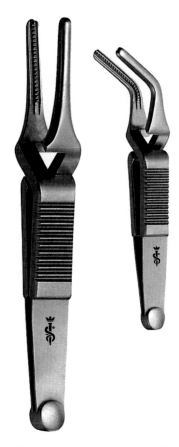

▣ Fig. 4.99 Mini Bulldog clamp. (Fa. Aesculap AG, with kind permission)

4.7 **Microsurgical Instruments**

Microsurgical instruments are used in many surgical departments in which work is performed under the microscope. They are particularly delicate and correspondingly sensitive to incorrect stress or improper use. For these instruments, other conditions apply in handling and presenting, instrument use and storage.

The instruments are constructed differently and are so finely built and ground that any incorrect use would damage the grinding or the tip. In the handles, the instruments are flattened or rounded and have a profile on the outside, which makes them safe to handle. If the handles are round, it is easy to rotate them during use without the need for a second hand. Some microsurgical instruments have a small cavity for the surgeon's fingers, so that the instrument can be used firmly and

4

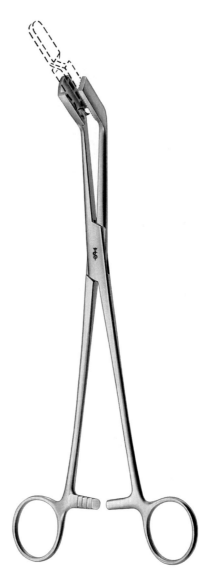

□ **Fig. 4.100** Forceps for replying and removing according to Johns-Hopkins. (Aesculap AG, with kind permission)

balanced, because under the microscope the view at the instrument is omitted, there must be felt surely whether the instrument lies well in the hand.

The forceps are anatomical, atraumatic or without grooves, but sharp forceps are also available. The scissors have a spring elastic mechanism and the needle holders are optionally available with or without ratchet.

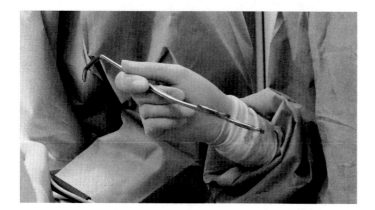

Fig. 4.101 Presenting a vascular clamp to clamp a vessel. (Photo by Margret Liehn)

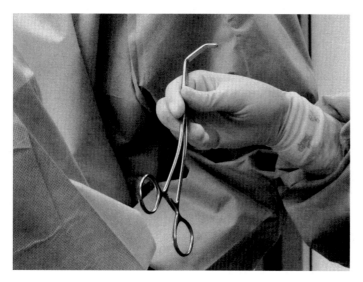

Fig. 4.102 Presenting a vascular clamp to clamp out a lumen. (Photo by Margret Liehn)

4

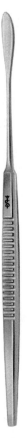

■ **Fig. 4.103**   Dissector according to Schmidt. (Aesculap AG, with kind permission)

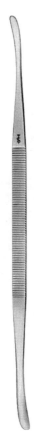

◨ **Fig. 4.104**   Dissector according to Tönnis. (Aesculap AG, with kind permission)

4

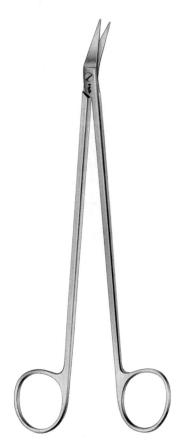

❑ Fig. 4.105   Angled scissors according to Potts de Martell. (Aesculap AG, with kind permission)

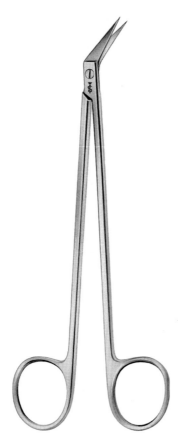

◻ **Fig. 4.106** Angled scissors according to De Bakey. (Aesculap AG, with kind permission)

4

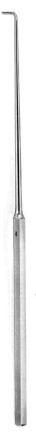

◘ **Fig. 4.107**   Nerve hook according to Crile. (Aesculap AG, with kind permission)

■ **Fig. 4.108** Nerve and vessel hook according to Caspar. (Aesculap AG, with kind permission)

4

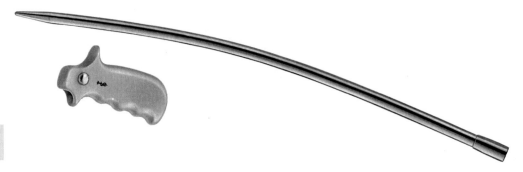

■ **Fig. 4.109**   Tunneling tube with handle according to Jenkner. (Aesculap AG, with kind permission)

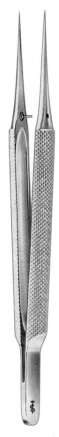

■ **Fig. 4.110**   Micro forceps with round handle. (Aesculap AG, with kind permission)

4.7.1   **Examples**

Examples of microsurgical instruments, shown in ■ Figs. 4.110, 4.111, 4.112, 4.113, and 4.114.

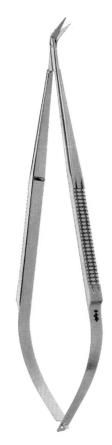

Fig. 4.111 Micro spring scissors with flat handle. (Aesculap AG, with kind permission)

■ **Handling**

Presenting microsurgical instruments under the microscope - view means placing and removing the instruments in such a way that the surgeon does not have to look away from the microscope. To do this, the instruments must be securely placed in the hand and removed again. Since the angle of approach varies with each operation and from surgeon to surgeon, it is necessary to practice how to approach the instrument without bumping into the microscope. Any jarring caused by uncontrolled bumping against the microscope will make the surgical site unrecognizable and will no longer allow accurate surgery. If instruments are in the situs at this moment, the risk of injury to the sensitive tissue is immense.

4

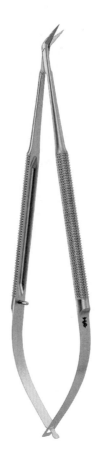

☐ Fig. 4.112   Micro spring scissors with round handle. (Aesculap AG, with kind permission)

On the instrument table, the fine instruments must be stored in such a way that they are not damaged. Rubber mats are available for this purpose, which provide support and protection for the instruments (☐ Fig. 4.115). Under no circumstances should their tips be bumped against the metal of the table because this will damage the covering material and thus sterility is no longer guaranteed and the tip of the instrument will be destroyed as well.

As a rule, microsurgical instruments, without ratchet too, are handed closed. The scrub nurse gently closes the instrument and presents it to the surgeon. The spring mechanism creates a slight pressure in the surgeons hand, which facilitates insertion into the small site. Only in exceptional cases, at the express request of the surgeon, can these instruments be handed open.

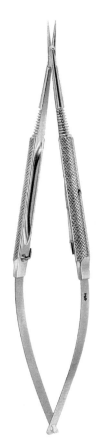

■ **Fig. 4.113** Microneedle holder with ratchet. (Aesculap AG, with kind permission)

Needle holders are available with and without ratchet. Here, too, it must be agreed with the surgeon whether the needle-thread combination is to be presented clamped or whether the needle holder is to be presented empty and the thread held separately under the microscope field so that the surgeon can clamp it himself. In the case of very thin material, the later option is to be preferred, as the needle is very difficult to see without an enlarging microscope.

For reprocessing, microsurgical instruments are also placed on rubber mats or fixed on suitable sieve trays, as they would be damaged by improper transport (▶ Sect. 7.3).

4

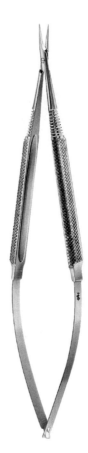

◘ **Fig. 4.114**   Microneedle holder without ratchet. (Aesculap AG, with kind permission)

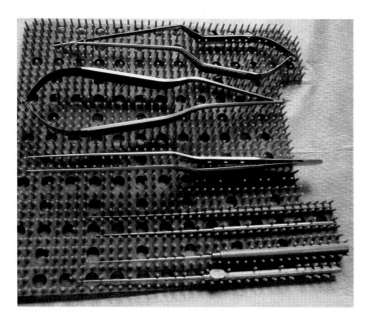

Fig. 4.115 Micro instruments on a rubber mat on the instrument table. (Photo by Margret Liehn)

The Instrument Table

In every operating theatre, there are standardised instrument-table setup instructions for the various procedures, which are binding for every employee. These standards are based on many rules. All instruments required for the planned intervention are prepared on the instrument table and the side table as well, in a standardized manner.

A good overview and a procedure-specific setup are important here (◻ Fig. 5.1).

The rule is to keep scalpels on the instrument table only as long as they are needed. As the covering materials are often available in a single layer, it must be borne in mind that scalpel blades must be protected separately so that they do not inadvertently penetrate the sterile covering material; a specially prepared towel should therefore be placed underneath. Anatomical dissection forceps are spatially separated from surgical sharp forceps, for example by scissors, so that there is no confusion. Placing tweezers inside each other to save space involves the risk of not being able to separate them when things have to be done quickly; in worst case then one tweezer falls down on the floor.

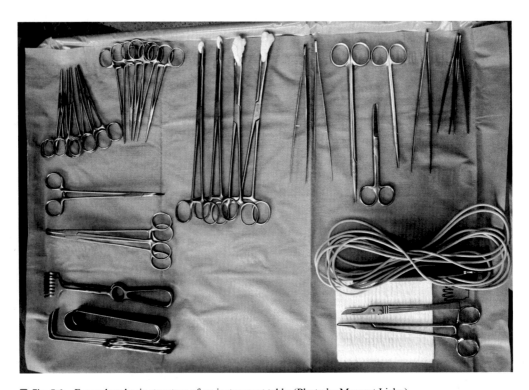

◻ **Fig. 5.1**   Exemplary basic structure of an instrument table. (Photo by Margret Liehn)

Retractors are prepared in pairs and the sharp hooks are always placed with the teeth facing upwards to avoid perforation of the sterile table cover. Often the sharp hooks are placed on the side table after opening the peritoneum.

Surgical sharp and anatomical dissection clamps are prepared in equal numbers according to standard. The department should agree whether an even or an odd number should always be placed on the instrument table. Different clamps are always placed in opposite directions on the table.

Scissors are prepared for organ preparation and for shortening the threads, the lengths depends on the operative situation.

Swabs are clamped in the straight dressing forceps, they are prepared in always the same number.

Instruments and clamped threads must never protrude or hang down over the edge of the table, as sterility cannot be guaranteed in this way. Only on the side of the instrument table facing the sterilely draped patient may the prepared swabs, for example, protrude over the edge of the table.

If liquids are required, there is a fixed code in the department for marking, which is binding for every employee. If required, there are small bowls with liquid on the instrument table, others on the side table.

Cable and electrode for the application of high-frequency current, suction hose with the appropriate attachment have to be applied with a self-adhesing strip at the sterile patient drapings.

If the suture material remains in the packaging until it is presented, the needle holder can be placed on the instrument table, making sure that the needle does not perforate the sterile table cover (◻ Fig. 5.2). As already mentioned with the scalpel blades, it is advisable to use a double cover for safety.

On the side tables, the instrument trays are placed next to each other in a sensible order. Sometimes it is necessary to stack trays one on top of the other, in which case the rule applies that all instruments normally required are taken out of the lower ones. Additional instruments that are sure to be needed can also be prepared on the instrument table. Anything that may be needed additionally is ready at hand on the side table(s) (◻ Fig. 5.3). All prepared, counted towels, suture materials, bowls for liquids and additionally required instruments have its place and are always within easy reach.

5

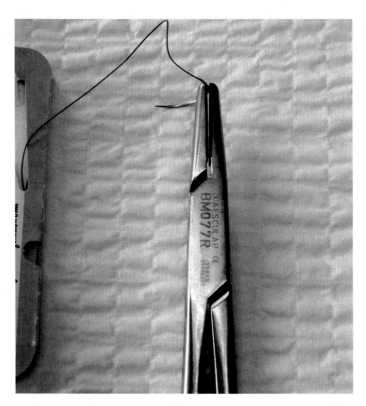

■ **Fig. 5.2** Prepared needle holder on the instrument table. An additional towel protects the table cover from perforation. (Photo by Margret Liehn)

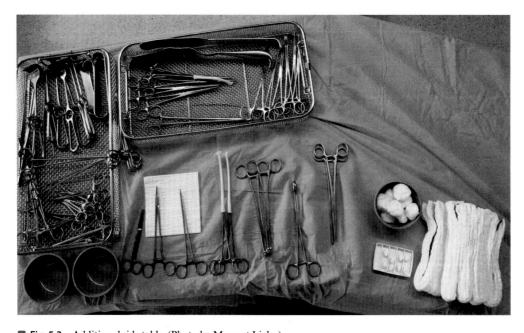

■ **Fig. 5.3**   Additional side table. (Photo by Margret Liehn)

Every employee uses the same table setup; after some time, each employee can find every instrument that is needed almost blindly without any effort. Every used instrument is put back in its original place to maintain overview, if necessary, after a superficial cleaning with a moist towel.

> Only after the count check and documentation of the count status of the instruments, swabs, towels and needles and after the skin suture has been completed the instruments may leave the OR-room to be reprocessed.

Handling of Surgical Instruments By the Scrub Nurse

Contents

© Springer-Verlag GmbH Germany, part of Springer Nature 2022
M. Liehn, H. Schlautmann, *101 of Surgical Instruments*, https://doi.org/10.1007/978-3-662-63632-9_6

In the description of the individual instruments, instructions on handling and presenting the instruments by the scrub nurse were given. Therefore, only the generally applicable guidelines are mentioned here.

Each instrument is grasped by the scrub nurse at the working part so that the surgeon can reach into the rings or around the handle and the instrument can be used immediately. The instrument lies straight or diagonally in the hand, depending on where and how it is needed in the situs.

Instruments with a curved or even double-curved working or gripping surface are difficult. Here, the scrub nurse must feel in advance how the instrument is used in order to correctly grasp the bend. The knowledge how the instrument will be used on the target organ is necessary . Everything changes when the surgeon is standing next to the scrub nurse or is left-handed. Anyhow, mistakes in handling at the beginning of training in the OR theatre can not be avoided and should not discourage the beginner.

Every scrub nurse must accompany the instrument with the eyes until the surgeon uses it, because this shows whether the presentation was correct. If the surgeon has to turn the instrument in the hand, the instrument – presentation must be critically reconsidered and corrected the next time.

Instruments with rings are generally held diagonally on the working part and are presented in such a way that the surgeon can reach into the rings. The exception is the dressing forceps with the clamped swab, which is held vertically (▶ Chap. 3, ◘ Fig. 3.34). Retractors are usually held horizontally as they are inserted into the surgical site. Forceps are held vertically.

Every sharp instrument, such as scalpels or sharp hooks, must be grasped from above so as not to endanger the scrub nurse during return.

The scrub nurse should always work with both hands. So it is possible to present the next instrument and take the removed one in one workflow. It makes sense to practice activities with the left hand (for right-handers) in order to achieve a certain degree of safety.

6.1   Getting Back the Used Instruments

In addition to the instrument presentation, the returning of the instruments is sometimes difficult to fit into the workflow. The used instrument is picked up with one hand, while the next instrument is ready in the other hand, so that the transition in the surgeon`s hand is smooth. Experienced nurses can receive an instrument with the splayed little finger and at the same time hand over a new instrument with the same hand. Scissors and tweezers required at the same time can also be handed over in this way, while an instrument is received with the second hand (► Chap. 3, ◘ Fig. 3.21).

Instruments are stained with blood when they are returned by the surgeon; blood corrodes the surface of the instruments if it is allowed to act for a longer time, and therefore the instruments are cleaned with a moisty towel by the scrub nurse; no NaCl is used for this purpose (► Chap. 7). In addition, blood-encrusted instruments stick to the gloves and cannot be used in an optimal way, scissor blades stick together, joints don`t work - all important reasons to clean an instrument after it has been removed and before it is placed on the instrument table in its standardized position. For cleaning, for example, a moist towel is used, which is not used on the patient.

The disposal of instruments at the end of a procedure takes place according to the rules of reprocessing (► Chap. 7) and begins during wound closure.

> Never instruments, towels and swabs leave the operating room until the procedure is complete and the count check has been finalized.

Reprocessing of Surgical Instruments

Contents

© Springer-Verlag GmbH Germany, part of Springer Nature 2022
M. Liehn, H. Schlautmann, *101 of Surgical Instruments*, https://doi.org/10.1007/978-3-662-63632-9_7

Since the surgical instruments of all surgical departments have an enormous financial value within the assets of a clinic, the function and value of the reusable medical devices must be maintained for many years by professional reprocessing. Several guidelines and legal regulations (for more informations: ► https://wfhss.com/links-2/, ► https://www.cdc.gov/), regulate the reprocessing by defined norms to make it transparent and to document the reprocessing procedures. The aim in reprocessing must be the preservation of value, efficiency ad hygiene.

Reprocessing in the form of cleaning, disinfection, checking, packaging, maintainment and sterilization takes place in the central department for sterile supply, hereinafter referred to as CSSD (central sterile supply department). An independent, highly technical department has emerged, whose employees have developed their own job description by qualified training.

Various institutions offer specialist courses in which participants are familiarized with the basics of instrument reprocessing. Certified standards are set by curricula.

The primary objective is to create a uniformly high-quality standard for the reprocessing of medical devices and provide tips and instructions for the practice of reprocessing.

There are working groups that repeatedly rethink and modify CSSD procedures. They determine guidelines, conditions and regulations for the reprocessing of medical devices, described in cooperation with the manufacturers.

7.1 Regulations

National, european or international guidelines are defined to make reprocessing processes comprehensible and to avoid damage to patients and staff.

7.2 Basic Rules

Basic requirement define that instruments should be reprocessed immediately after use, if possible, so that blood and other contaminants do not dry on and in the instruments, as this makes cleaning and disinfection more difficult. It also requires that instruments be disassembled into their individual parts, if necessary, so that all surfaces are accessible to the disinfectant (e.g. ISO 176442004 has been prepared by technical Committee CENT/TC 204 "Sterilization of medical devices" which is held by BSI (British Standards Institution). (for more informations: ► https://www.bsigroup.com).

Unused instruments must also be reprocessed in the same way as used instruments, i.e. they must be disassembled and/or opened.

Factory new instruments and instruments from repair returns must undergo the entire reprocessing process according to the manufacturer's instructions before being used for the first time.

7.2.1 Use in the Operating Theatre

A so-called instrument cycle, defined by a German organization for instrument reprocessing, begins with use in the operating room.

Instrument cycle
- Use
- Dismantling
- Cleaning
- Disinfection
- Optical inspection
- Maintenance (functional test)
- Sterilization (documentation)
- Storage (provision for use)

■ **Surgical Instruments in Use**

During surgery, instruments should not come into contact with saline solution (NaCl), as after prolonged contact on stainless steel instruments the solution attacks the surface and corrosion can occur. Unfortunately, this often cannot be avoided intraoperatively. Iodine solution, skin and mucous membrane disinfectants and some lubricants attack the surfaces of the instruments and make subsequent reprocessing of the instruments more difficult.

Likewise, proper use of surgical instruments according to their intended purpose during the surgical procedure is of great importance for maintaining the value of the instruments. Used instruments after ending the surgical procedure must be correctly half-opened and dismantled and placed on a standardized, machine-suitable tray to prevent damage to the instruments. The carbide inserts on scissors or needle holders can split off, and if more delicate instruments come to lie under the heavy ones, deformation will occur.

7

After the contaminated instruments have been deposited on standardized trays, they are cleaned and disinfected in the cleaning-disinfection machine. In many cases, these trays have the name of the used tray or a defined number to facilitate assignment by the CSSD staff. Based on the name or number, the instruments can be returned to the respective tray by means of documentation. The trays must not be overloaded, as otherwise effective rinsing of all parts is not guaranteed, resulting in so-called rinsing shadows. Heavy instruments should be placed at the bottom or on the side of the trays, vessels and bowls should be placed with the opening facing downwards so that no cleaning water can collect, this supports the subsequent drying process.

All instruments that have joints (e.g. scissors, clamps, forceps, needle holders) must be placed in a half-open position in order to make e.g. blood in the ratchets and jaws accessible for disinfection and cleaning. When closed, blood and secrete cannot be removed and the instrument remains contaminated. The joints should be opened as soon as the instruments are put down in order to prevent additional stress and risk to the CSSD staff. Instruments that can be disassembled should be deposited in individual trays.

In order to prevent damage, mats suitable for dishwashers should be used for fine instruments.

Requirements for OR Staff for the Disposal of Instruments

- For reusable scalpel handles, the scalpel blade must be removed from the handle.
- To avoid injury, a clamp should be used for removal.
- Needles and other sharp objects must be disposed of in appropriate safety boxes.
- High-frequency cables and motor systems are placed in the special tray in an orderly fashion (❑ Fig. 7.1).
- Motor systems are arranged on separate holding devices, compressed air hoses can be plugged together and can thus be prepared mechanically.
- Microsurgical instruments are placed on special mats.
- MIS instruments are disassembled according to the manufacturer's instructions.
- Optics must be protected from impact and shock (the manufacturer provides appropriate storage racks).
- Waste and residues of disinfectants must not be placed in the disposal tray.

The instruments are to be disposed in the operating area in a standardized manner so that the employees of the CSSD have as little contact as possible with the contaminated instruments.

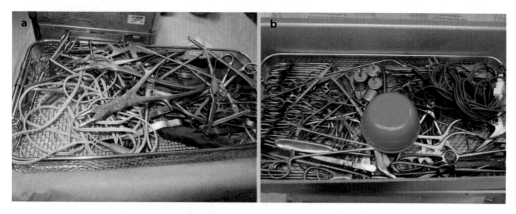

□ **Fig. 7.1** **a, b** Incorrect **a** and correct **b** disposal of instruments and high-frequency cables. (Photo by Margret Liehn)

7.2.2 Disposal

Dry disposal of used instrument trays is preferable to wet disposal.

Advantages of Dry Disposal
- Low weight of the disposal containers.
- No risk of corrosion on the surface alloy.
- Low costs, as neither disinfectant nor water is required here.
- No foam formation in the cleaning-disinfection machine.
- Environmental friendly.

Disadvantages of Dry Disposal
- If you wait too long for reprocessing, there is a risk of corrosion on the instruments due to the effect of various rinsing solutions and the patient's body fluids on the surface of the instruments.

■ **Advantages of Wet Disposal**
Advantages are not known.

The instruments are placed in the tray in dedicated disposal containers (hard or soft packaging) and sealed. Depending on the organization of a clinic, the used instruments are transported in a container trolley to the unclean side of the CSSD (□ Fig. 7.2).

7.3 Reprocessing in the CSSD

When procuring new medical devices, care must be taken to ensure that the instruments, tubing systems, endoscopic instruments, motors, straight and angled handpieces can be repro-

7

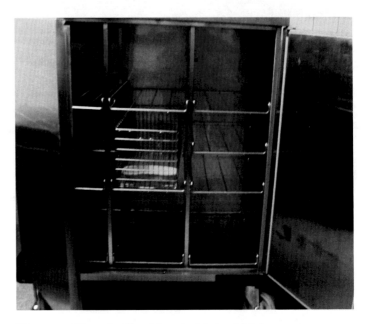

◘ Fig. 7.2   Disposal trolley. (Photo by Margret Liehn)

cessed by machine. Instruments that can be disassembled are preferable to those that cannot. In this case, the manufacturer's instructions must be followed, otherwise, the warranty may be voided.

According to guidelines, special attention must be paid to the number of reprocessing cycles. Due to the very frequent use of the instruments, increased attention must be paid to wear and tear of the products, in particular to the brittleness of the material and alterations of the surfaces. Here, the manufacturer must fix a limitation of reprocessing cycles and the user must observe this.

Permanent training of the staff in the handling of the materials, also by the instrument manufacturers, ensures a long service life of the instruments.

7.3.1   Cleaning and Disinfection

The procedure for manual reprocessing must also be defined in standardized work instructions. All critical steps must be evaluated by means of risk analysis, the success of the cleaning must be ensured by means of validation and regularly be checked.

Machine reprocessing is always preferable to manual reprocessing.

- **Manual Reprocessing**
- Disinfectant solutions for manual reprocessing are applied.
- Never warm disinfectant solution above room temperature.
- Instruments are first disinfected and then cleaned. Combined solutions are used here, which both clean and disinfect; protein fixation must not be provoked. The manufacturer's instructions must be observed when using the products with regard to concentration and contact time.
- The solutions must be renewed daily, as prolonged use leads to a risk of corrosion due to contamination and evaporation of the solution (increased concentration) as well as a decrease in the disinfection effect due to increased contamination.
- The instruments must be completely wetted with the disinfectant solution.
- Do not use metal brushes or scouring agents for manual cleaning, as these destroy the surface of the instruments.
- After chemical disinfection, all instruments must be rinsed intensively with clear running and fully demineralized (deionized) water. The instruments are then dried immediately.

- **Ultrasonic Cleaning**

Ultrasound propagates in the water at certain frequencies. This effect is used in the ultrasonic cleaning of surgical instruments. An ultrasonic basin is filled with fully demineralized water. A disinfectant can be added as required (◻ Fig. 7.3).

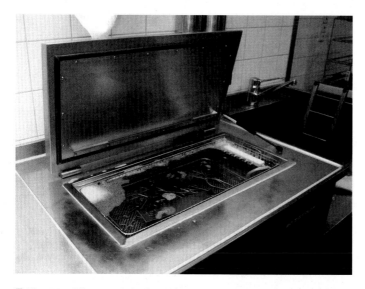

◻ **Fig. 7.3** Ultrasound basin. (CSSD Marienhospital Osnabrück, with kind permission)

The device generates an ultrasonic field in the liquid. The resulting vibrations lead to the formation of bubbles (cavitations), which condense explosively on surfaces. The resulting pressure waves cause friction and the dirt particles are mechanically loosened in and on the instruments.

This procedure is used for mechanical support during manual cleaning or pre-treatment of instruments with dried-on soiling prior to machine cleaning.

After each ultrasonic cleaning, the instruments must be mechanically rinsed with fully demineralized water and then dried.

Note: Microsurgical instruments should not be treated by ultrasound!

■ Mechanical Cleaning and Disinfection

When cleaning the instruments by machine, care must be taken to ensure that the pre-cleaning is carried out with cold water, as protein clumping (denaturation) occurs at temperatures above 40 °C and the instruments become encrusted.

Only in the event of an epidemic is disinfection carried out first, followed by cleaning.

Checklists are used to check the cleaning-disinfection machines before they are put into operation:
— Check the flushing arms and the flushing nozzles,
— Check the fine and coarse lint screens,
— Check the connections and the charging trolley,
— Visual inspection of the interior and exterior (silica can cause discoloration of the instruments),
— Check whether cleaning additives are present.
— If possible, control the supply of demineralized water.

Due to thermal disinfection, no disinfectant is required. The cleaning and disinfecting machine must be loaded in such a way that all instruments can completely be rinsed and the rinsing arms are not blocked. Validation of the mentioned cleaning procedure must correspond to the current state of science and technology.

■ Special Requirement for MIS Instruments

The MIS instruments are made of different materials:
— Chrome and chrome-nickel steel,
— Non-ferrous metal alloys, e.g. chromium-plated brass,
— Anodized aluminum,
— Plastics and plastic-coated metals,
— Glass in the optics.

Due to the narrow lumens and difficult-to-access areas on the MIS instruments, the chemical products used must ensure optimal cleaning and at the same time act mild on the material.

Following the manufacturer's instructions, the instruments are disassembled, the seals removed, the taps opened and placed on a cleaning machine insert specially designed for these instruments. The tubular instruments with their taps opened are connected to flushing hoses in the cleaning machine so that flushing of the tubes is guaranteed.

For endoscopic instruments, the industry offers special endoscopy-cleaning and disinfecting machines, which clean the sensitive instruments on a chemical-thermal basis.

7.3.2 Maintenance and Functional Testing

Disinfection and cleaning of the instruments are followed by visual inspection, maintenance and technical testing. Each instrument is taken individually and checked macroscopically for cleanliness, drying condition, integrity, function and completeness. To avoid metallic abrasion, the instrument must have cooled down before the functional test. It is to check whether the joints are in good working order and whether the instrument is free of damage. If damaged, the instrument must be sent for repair.

The following damage, among others, can occur to an instrument:

- **Flash rust**: Fine iron dust produced by abrasion rusts in the air and settles on other instruments (◻ Fig. 7.4).
- **Stress cracks**: occur in cases where the instrument is exposed to high stresses due to its design, e.g. at the rivet and screw connections of the grasping forceps. For this reason, the instruments must be cleaned in an open state. If they are to be sterilized in the locked state, they must be fixed in the first ratchet (◻ Fig. 7.5).

After cleaning, all instruments on which friction occurs during use (joints, clasps, detents) require special care. To ensure that the instruments can be used permanently, they must be lubricated. The lubricant may only be applied to that points where friction occurs on the instrument. Excess must be removed with a lint-free cloth.

Example of the Functional Test of a Shear

Depending on the design of the scissors, various test materials can be selected for testing the cutting surfaces: Gauze ban-

7

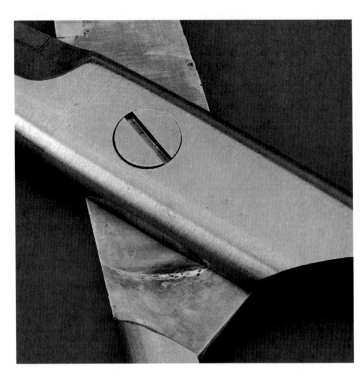

◰ **Fig. 7.4** Corrosion in the joint area of a shear. (From: "Instrument reprocessing done right" Instrument Reprocessing Working Group, with kind permission AKI (Aus: »Instrumentenaufbereitung richtig gemacht« Arbeitskreis Instrumentenaufbereitung, mit freundlicher Genehmigung))

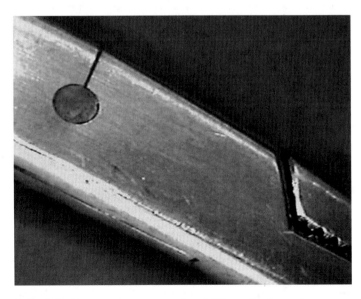

◰ **Fig. 7.5** Stress crack on a screw thread. (From: "Instrument reprocessing done right" Instrument Reprocessing Working Group, with kind permission AKI (Aus: »Instrumentenaufbereitung richtig gemacht« Arbeitskreis Instrumentenaufbereitung, mit freundlicher Genehmigung))

dage, cotton or rayon compresses. It is recommended not to apply lateral pressure on the branches during the cutting test (make 3 uninterrupted cuts):

- Cut should be oblique and transverse to the weaving ribs.
- The scissors must not get caught when cutting.
- The test material must not fray or tear.
- 2/3 of the blade length must cut.

If the blades are impeccable, the scissors can be returned to instrument cycle. If the scissors are dull or the joints are stiff, they must be sent to an authorized dealer or directly to the instrument manufacturer for instrument repair.

All modern CSSD departments have a database in which all instruments, as well as all instrument trays from all departments of a clinic, are saved. Only with good cooperation between the surgical department and the CSSD is it possible to maintain this instrument database. All changes to the trays must be communicated with the CSSD.

With the help of the developed packing lists for the individual surgical trays, the instruments can be sorted back into the trays in a standardized manner based on the article number. Each department has individual packing lists, but basic rules determine that retractors are placed together, clamps and scissors are sorted according to size and length. These steps are followed by packing.

7.3.3 Packing

The following requirements must be met by the packaging:
- It must be possible to pack the materials without problems before sterilization.
- Each packaging must be adapted to the respective sterilization process.
- Sterile storage must be guaranteed with the packaging.

To ensure that sterility is maintained until the next use, sterile goods must be protected from moisture, dust and the ingress of germs.

- **Packaging Options**
- Disposable packaging
- Sterilization paper (in combination with towels for heavy single instruments), cotton cloths are to be avoided!
- Film (a combination of paper and film for single instruments): Paper packaging is considered soft packaging, is disposable and not reusable.

- Reusable packaging
- Aluminium containers: Container systems are considered to be hard packaging that is stackable, break-proof and reusable.

The packaging shall provide the user with the following information
- Contents (e.g. basic tray, Orthopedic tray),
- Type of sterilization (steam, gas or plasma sterilization),
- Sterilization date,
- Expiration Date,
- Label number (enables traceability of the reprocessing process in case of incidents).

The instrument tray is first wrapped in a cloth or paper according to defined standards and then packed in the container or another sheet of paper. The cloth and paper are folded in such a way that the circulating nurse can easily open the package under sterile conditions without reaching over the sterile instrument (◘ Fig. 7.6).

The inner packaging of the container or even the paper packaging has great influence on the sterilization result. Wrapping the trays, preferably in a cloth (e.g. lint-free cloth made of blended fabric), supports drying within the sterilization container or the outer paper packaging and thus minimizes residual moisture and the risk of corrosion.

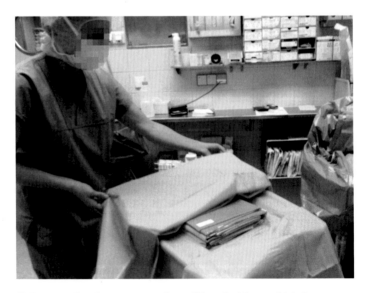

◘ **Fig. 7.6** Opening a paper package. (Photo by Margret Liehn)

Preserved sterility depends essentially on the handling and storage conditions for the sterile goods. After the checked and technically flawless instruments are in their respective packaging, they are sealed:
- Containers are closed with a lid and sealed.
- Instrument trays are wrapped in a cloth and a sheet of paper.
- Transparent bags and tubes as well as paper bags are sealed with a film sealer.

The materials are then labeled:
- Designation of the object (e.g. basic tray, Luer forceps, hammer),
- Name of the employee who packed the instruments/items,
- Sterilization date,
- Expiration date,
- Type of sterilization (steam, gas, plasma sterilization).

The containers are placed on a sterilization trolley, the individual instruments are placed in a rack in such a way that sterilization is ensured and placed in the autoclave (◘ Fig. 7.7).

There should be a standard that describes the correct loading of the autoclave.

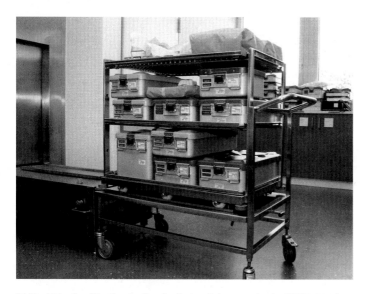

◘ **Fig. 7.7** Sterilization trolley (in front of the autoclave). (CSSD Marienhospital Osnabrück, with kind permission)

7.3.4 Sterilization

Sterilization is a process by which remaining microorganisms on the instruments are killed. The procedures of sterilization, just like the reprocessing procedures, should be defined by standardized validation procedures and guidelines.

■ **Sterilization Process**

The following are the sterilization procedures commonly used in a clinic.

■ **Steam Sterilization**

In steam sterilization, pure saturated steam is used to heat the sterilization chamber to 121 °C or 134 °C. This temperature is maintained with moist heat for a prescribed time. This is followed by a drying phase. The instruments (134 °C) or rubber materials (121 °C) should come out of the sterilizer completely dry at the end of sterilization. The loading weight is 10 kg and should not be exceeded. If the trays are moist, the process must be repeated or a technician must check the equipment.

Steam sterilization can be performed on all thermostable (heat-resistant) materials, i.e. the materials must not be altered by either the heat or the vacuum. The manufacturer's instructions must be observed. It must be ensured that the steam has access to the material at all points.

Advantages of steam sterilization
- cost-effective,
- environmental friendly,
- non-toxic,
- controllable,
- there are no residues on the materials (stains).

The following materials can be steam-sterilized:
- stainless steel,
- textiles,
- rubber products,
- heat-resistant plastic.

After the sterilization process, the sterile material must be "dry".

■ **Low Temperature Sterilization**

These procedures are used for heat-sensitive (thermolabile) materials. The manufacturer's instructions must be observed. These sterilization variants are useful for:

- heat-sensitive probes,
- optics,
- flexible endoscopes.

The manufacturer's instructions must be observed.

■ **Gas Sterilization**

There are two options here:
- Gas sterilization with ethylene oxide (EO),
- Gas sterilization with formaldehyde (FO).
- Gas sterilization with **ethylene oxide**
    - Here, at low temperatures (approx. 55 °C) and high humidity (70%), toxic gas denaturizes the proteins of the germs.
    - Since EO is highly toxic and must not remain in the material, only the manufacturer can determine the specific sterile airing time required to remove all toxic gases.
- Gas sterilization with **formaldehyde**
    - Formaldehyde denaturizes the germs and the proteins. Here, the steam in the sterilization chamber is heated to 55–65 °C and the sterile material is moistened. Then 3% formaldehyde is added. At 100% relative humidity, the gas can act on germs and protein. The exposure time is 60 min.
    - Since FO settles on the materials, the materials must be aired out after the sterilization process according to the manufacturer's instructions.

■ **Plasma Sterilization**

This process can also be used to sterilize highly labile instruments and immediately return them to the instrument circuit. Here, hydrogen peroxide is used to kill the microorganisms by means of free radicals (highly active compounds that destroy microorganisms) at a chamber temperature of 45 °C. Proper instructions in the handling of the device is necessary. The advantage of this procedure is the short, toxin-free sterilization time.

Unfortunately, the costs for plasma sterilizers are very high, in addition, there are costs for required special wrapping paper.

■ **Sterility Control**

All sterilizers must be checked for effectiveness before being put into operation. A daily **test** on the steam sterilizer verifies that the air has been adequately pumped out before introducing the steam. Without a vacuum, the steam saturation will not reach the correct concentration.

Before loading the sterilization trolleys, all materials are scanned for documentation. After completion of all sterilization processes, the batch documentation is used to check whether the sterilization processes were performed in a proper condition (example: ◻ Table 7.1). The sterilization process contains the following parameters:

- Temperature,
- Pressure,
- Sterilization time.

The release of the sterile items is one of the most important sub-processes in the reprocessing of medical devices, since in this sub-step the decision must be made whether the sterile items can be used on the patient or not. The approval may only be carried out by persons who have obtained the authorization through qualification and further training.

In the event of error messages during sterilization, the entire process must be repeated. Quality management is

◻ **Table 7.1**   Standard for the release of sterile goods (CSSD of the Marienhospital Osnabrück, with kind permission)

Indication	Action	Note
After every batch		
Control of the packaging	The packaging must be checked for damage and moisture	In the event of damaged packaging, residual moisture, the sterile items must be repackaged and sterilized, including changing the container inner packaging and the disposable filter
Control of the loading and the batch record in the EDP	Control of the course curve Control of the individual process parameters	The batch must be repeated in the event of error messages
Control of the barcode labels	Compare the current barcode label number with the batch record	If the barcode number is missing, the sterile goods must be released using manual batch comparison in the EDP
Release	Approval is to be carried out by EDP	

Note: This document was reviewed by Mr. Dr. Gross on 21.10.2019 and was reviewed by the Hygiene Commission on 14/11/2019 released!

required for monitoring reprocessing in a CSSD, which can stand up to external scrutiny at any time. In the event of damage (e.g. infection) to the patient, the clinic must prove that all processes in the clinic were carried out properly.

After completion of the sterilization process, the sterilization trolley is pulled out of the sterilization chamber. After the sterilized material has cooled down, the materials on the (clean) sterilized side are returned to the instrument cycle. For this purpose, the instruments are either kept in the CSSD or returned to the function areas. In preparation for the surgical procedure, the employee in the department finds a technically flawless, sterile set of instruments.

The prerequisite for the protected storage of sterile items is a dust-free and dry environment. To protect the instruments from corrosion, the environment should also not be exposed to temperature fluctuations. These conditions allow a storage time of up to 6 months or longer.

Supplementary Information

Further Reading – 224

© Springer-Verlag GmbH Germany, part of Springer Nature 2022
M. Liehn, H. Schlautmann, *101 of Surgical Instruments*, https://doi.org/10.1007/978-3-662-63632-9

Further Reading

Arbeitskreis Instrumentenaufbereitung (2012) Instrumentenaufbereitung richtig gemacht. 10. überarbeitete Auflage. http://www.a-k-i.org/ (frei zugängliches pdf; letzter Zugriff: 01.11.2016)

Braun Aesculap. Instruments4you. http://www.instruments4you.de; letzter Zugriff: 13.03.2021

Carus T (2009) Operationsatlas laparoskopische Chirurgie. Springer, Berlin Heidelberg

Carus T (2014) Operationsatlas Laparoskopische Chirurgie, 3rd edn. Springer, Berlin Heidelberg, New York

Liehn M, Grüning S, Köhnsen N (2006) OP und Anästhesie. Springer, Berlin Heidelberg

Liehn M, Lengersdorf B, Steinmüller L, Döhler R (2016) OP-Handbuch, 6th edn. Springer, Berlin Heidelberg

Liehn M, Steinmüller L, Döhler R (2011) OP-Handbuch, 5th edn. Springer, Berlin Heidelberg

Liehn M, Lengersdorf B, Steinmüller L, Döhler R (2020) OP-Handbuch, 7th edn. Springer, Berlin Heidelberg

Wintermantel E, Suk-Woo H (2009) Medizintechnik Life science engineering, 5th edn. Springer, Berlin Heidelberg, New York

With the friendly support of

Klaus Dieter Harmel (Niels Stensen Clinics Marienhospital Osnabrück, Ltd. CSSD)

Manuela Junker (Niels Stensen Clinics Marienhospital Osnabrück) Gabriele Frank

All employees of the OR theatre of the Asklepios Klinik Altona (AKA)

Printed in the United States
by Baker & Taylor Publisher Services